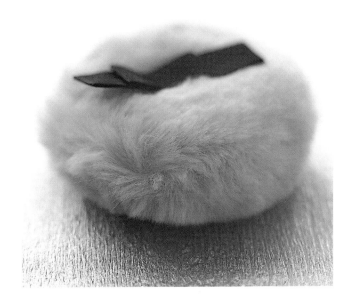

timeless
beauty

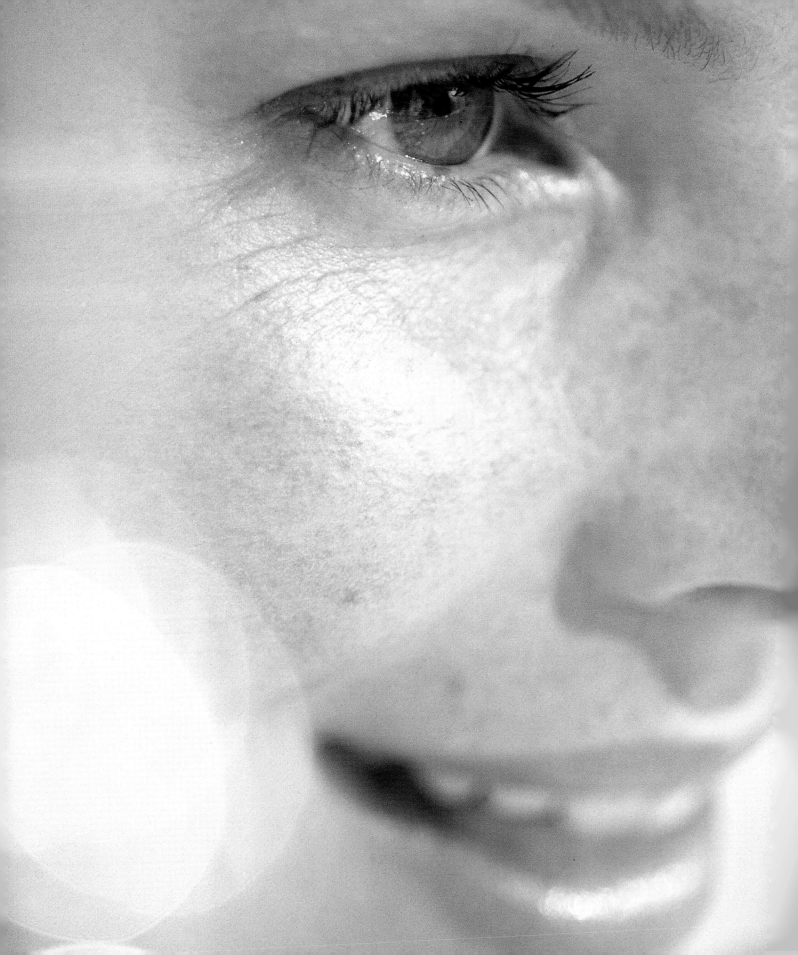

Good Housekeeping

timeless
beauty

look and feel ten years younger

Jo Glanville-Blackburn

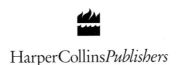

HarperCollins*Publishers*

First published in 2001 by

HarperCollins*Publishers*

77–85 Fulham Palace Road

London W6 8JB

The HarperCollins website address is:

www.**fire**and**water**.com

05 04 03 02 01 00

9 8 7 6 5 4 3 2 1

Published in association with The National Magazine
Company Limited. Good Housekeeping is a registered
trade mark of The National Magazine Company Limited.

The Good Housekeeping website address is:
www.goodhousekeeping.com

The expression Good Housekeeping as used in the title of
the book is the mark of the National Magazine Company
Limited and the Hearst Corporation, registered in the
United Kingdom and the USA, and other principal
countries in the world, and is the absolute property of
the National Magazine Company and the Hearst
Corporation. The use of this trade mark other than with
the express permission of the National Magazine
Company Limited or the Hearst Corporation is strictly
prohibited.

Copyright © 2001 HarperCollins*Publishers*/The National
Magazine Company Limited

A CIP catalogue record for this book is available from the
British Library.

ISBN: 0 00 713116 X

Colour reproduction by Colourscan, Singapore
Printed and bound in the UK by Bath Press

This book is typeset in HelveticaNeue and
Simoncini Garamond

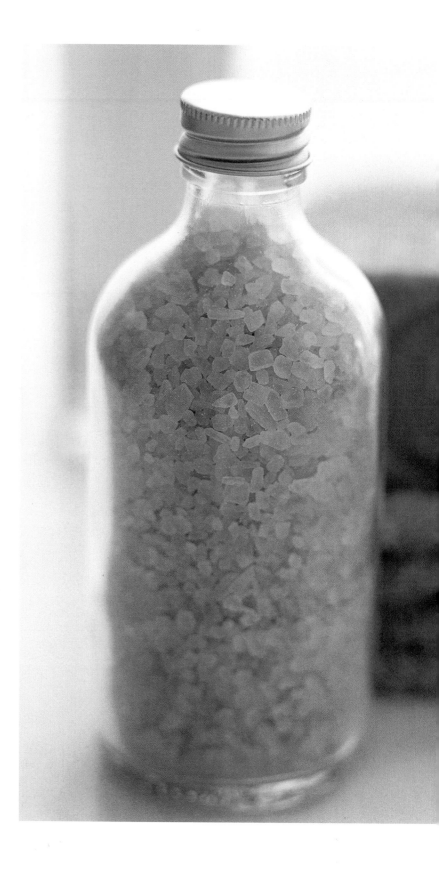

contents

foreword

This is the age of anti-ageing and there's never been a time quite like it. We don't just have choices – we're deluged with advice. Our only problem is, what exactly to opt for. Thankfully, we've graduated from the 'duty to be beautiful' era of faddy, costly, obsessional regimes. We now know from experience that the best, most intelligent beauty systems fit into our lifestyles seamlessly – they suit the way we want to look and feel by saving valuable time, yet giving us sensual satisfaction.

At the end of the day, looking great should be a matter of good, creative fun with a healthy dose of self-indulgence calculated in. That's why this book is such a great guide. While sorting good, practical fact from fluffy beauty fiction (and let's face it, there's still enough of that around), it provides inspiration for grown-up women to exploit their sexy, sassy individuality to the full.

Whether you're a baby boomer on the brink of a challenging new life phase or a thirty-something searching for a look good, feel great gameplan you really can call an investment, this is the expert reference you'll dip into again and again to fulfil your needs. Most of all, it's a rich and easy source of achievable tips and pointers that with practise, become second nature. And isn't that the blueprint of timeless beauty? At *Good Housekeeping* we believe it is – and we've more than a hunch you do too. Enjoy yourselves!

Vicci Bentley, Beauty Director
Good Housekeeping

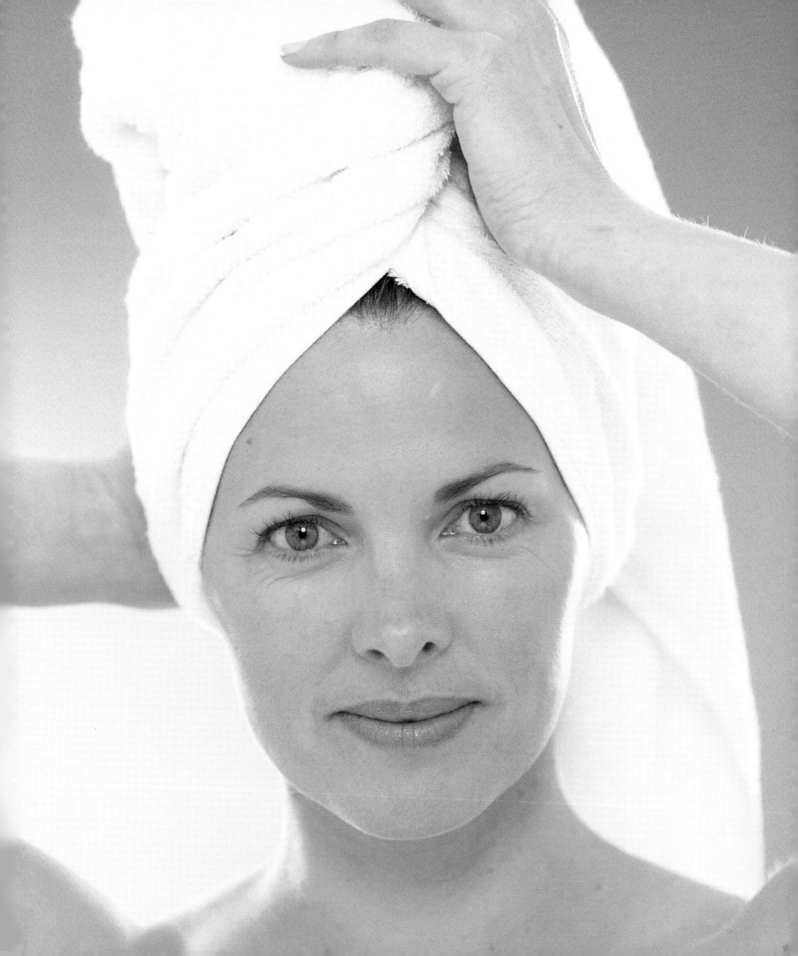

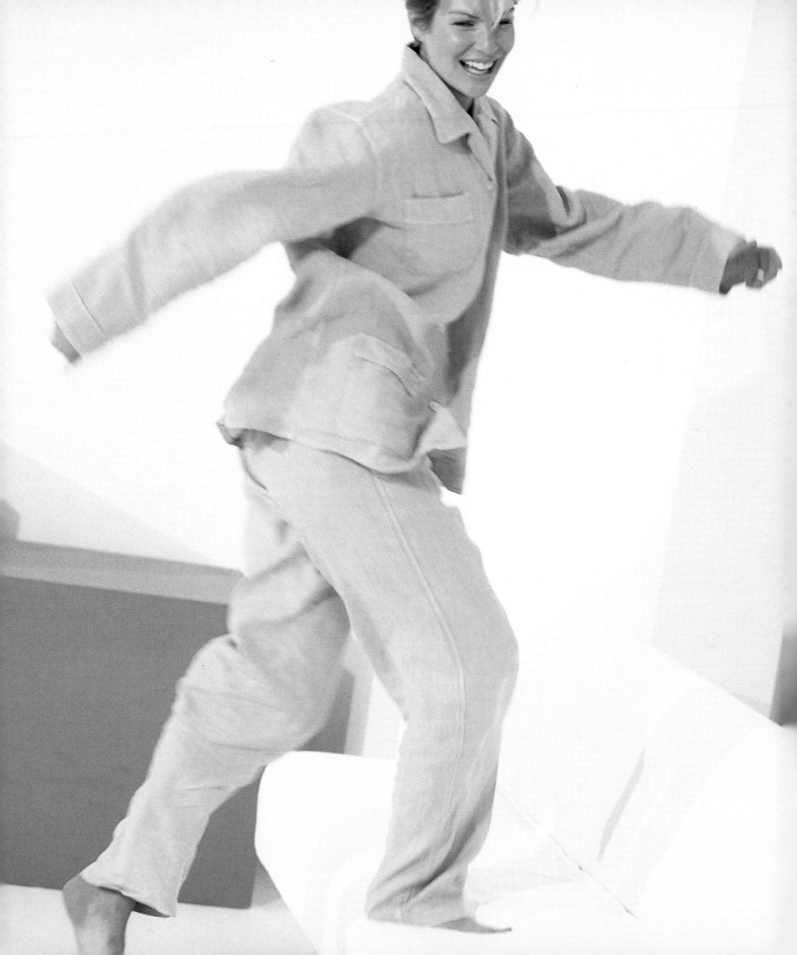

know yourself

Timeless Beauty is about a developing a passion for living and enjoying your life to the full. When you feel positive and happy, you exude energy, enthusiasm and true beauty without any need for cosmetic help. It's my belief that happiness really does make you look as good as you feel, and those around you can see it in your face and the way you carry yourself.

Why timeless? Because beauty exists at every age. It's not about youth and perfection, it's about knowing yourself: developing inner confidence and self-assurance that make you look your very best, whatever your age.

Timeless Beauty is top-to-toe beauty – made easy. It's designed to appeal to women of all ages and offer a more positive and better understanding of ourselves as we begin the ageing processes. It also offers very real advice on how to keep your skin, hair, body, make-up and even your spirits fresh and vibrant, with tips and tricks that consistently work rather than simply following a fashion.

It has been designed to fit in with your lifestyle, too. There are time-saving solutions throughout for all of us who lead a hectic life but still need to make time for ourselves; and more in-depth regimes for times when we can afford to indulge ourselves that little bit more.

I hope you find it useful over many years to come.

Jo Glanville-Blackburn

your skin

soft, sensitive and sensual

to the touch, your skin

surrounds and protects

millions of nerve endings

that bring the flush of

youth and the radiance

of life to your looks

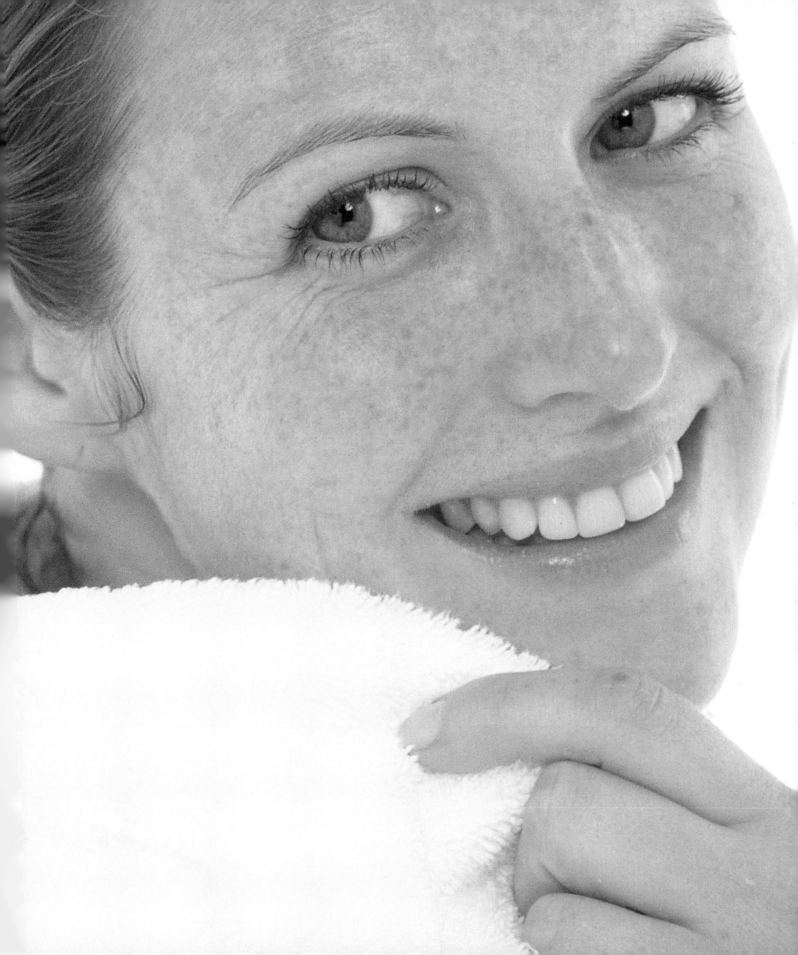

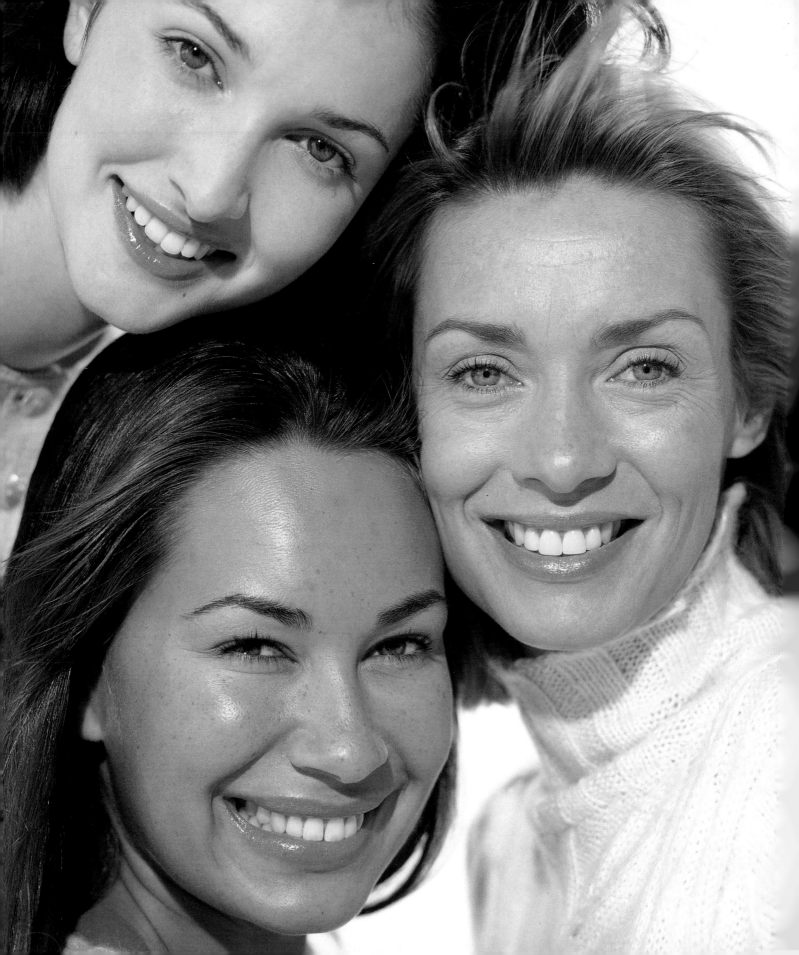

how and why skin ages

what's going on

The way we treat our skin has a dramatic effect as we get older. In our 20s it didn't seem to matter, but things slow down with age and lack of care soon becomes apparent.

Young skin is plump, vital and renews itself every 28 days, requiring little or no help to do so. However, as we age, everything slows down. Fewer oils are produced, so skin feels drier; cell renewal takes longer, so the skin's surface layer (the protective barrier) allows crucial amounts of moisture out; and the collagen and elastin fibres that support the skin and keep it looking firm and wrinkle-free begin to sag and bag until skin looks thin and crepey. Just how your skin ages is partly pre-ordained by your genes – you only need to look at your parents to get a fairly good idea of what to expect. However, this only accounts for around 20 per cent of lines and wrinkles: the rest is down to your lifestyle. The good news is that we now know so much more about how different lifestyles age the body and the skin that you can aim to improve the odds and look better at 50 and beyond than your mother ever did.

in your 20s

Your skin is supple and elastic, quick to heal and relatively wrinkle-free. You may experience the occasional breakout or oiliness, but by your mid to late 20s, hormones and oil production will be almost totally balanced. There is evidence that collagen and elastin are able to regenerate themselves as long as they are protected from UV light and pollution.

golden rules of the 20s

■ **Protect your skin** daily from UV light and pollution as early as possible. Experts insist that damage prevention at this age is the most vital anti-ageing skincare tactic there is.

■ **Establish your skincare routine now.** Start regular cleansing, toning and moisturising twice a day. Ensure that you always remove your make-up thoroughly before bed, and drink plenty of mineral water.

■ **Don't neglect your diet** and try to find time to relax. Late nights partying can wreak havoc with your skin. You can only feed your skin from the inside, and a bad diet will show itself in your skin first.

in your 30s

Your skin probably looks great and, if you act now, it will stay looking its best for as long as possible. The colour and tone of your face, neck and chest may appear slightly uneven – this is due to skin pigment cells becoming less efficient at producing skin colour. If you have been a sun worshipper during your teens and 20s, exposure to sunlight will have reduced your skin's elasticity, leading to a few premature wrinkles. By now you've probably noticed those fine lines that have started to appear around the corners of your eyes and along your forehead.

golden rules in your 30s

■ **Always wear a high protection sunscreen** on your face, backs of hands and chest. Invest more in your daily moisturiser (perhaps one incorporating UV protection). And look for creams containing antioxidants, as free-radical damage speeds up now, resulting in drier skin and patchy, uneven pigmentation.

■ **Pay special attention to the delicate skin around your eyes** – the first place to show signs of wrinkles – and to your hands and décolleté.

■ **Exfoliate sensibly.** Cell renewal is beginning to slow down, so regular exfoliation plays an essential role in removing dead skin cells, which make skin look dull, from the skin's surface. Creams containing exfoliating alpha-hydroxy acids (AHA) can make a real difference.

■ **Don't try to skimp on your vitamin intake.** Your 30s can be very demanding: you may be juggling a career with children. Make sure you are getting the nutrients your body, and your skin, needs. Top up with additional iron, vitamin-B complex, vitamins C and E and evening primrose oil. These are all vital supplements for women.

in your 40s

It is likely that your skin will begin losing its elasticity, smile and frown lines will deepen, crow's feet at the corners of your eyes will look more pronounced, and age spots may become more defined. This is because there is less fat padding under your skin, which in turn may produce thinner looking lips and more pronounced, gaunt-looking cheekbones. But it's not all bad news – you can appear more radiant and self-assured because you are more confident about yourself. And now is the time to reduce any kind of stress in your life: this always shows in your skin first.

golden rules of your 40s

■ **Moisturising remains a top priority.** Switch to a richer cream, invest in a regular facial and more specific skincare treatments for other parts of your body, particularly the neck and hands.

■ **Be gentle with your skin.** Recent research suggests that over-zealous exfoliating in your 40s and beyond thins the skin's protective outer layer almost too much, so that harmful UV is able to penetrate deeper, faster.

■ **Stay out of the sun.** The continual decline in your skin's production of melanin makes changes in skin pigmentation even more dramatic, so increase your SPF levels and avoid sun exposure. Age spots, otherwise known as sun spots, are caused by sun damage accumulated from years of UV exposure.

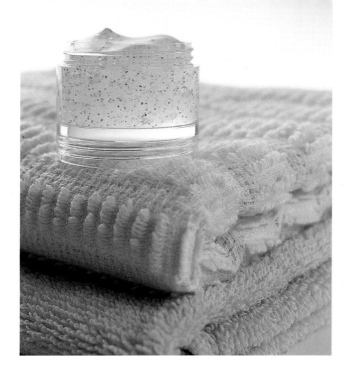

in your 50s and beyond

After the menopause, skin takes longer to renew itself due to the slowing down of the amounts of oestrogen we produce. The surface of the skin holds less moisture, oil gland activity slows down so skin feels naturally drier, and lines becomes more noticeable, not just around the eyes but around the mouth, the cheeks and the throat too. The deposits of collagen underneath your skin have shrunk, so you experience more sagging, usually around the jawline.

As your oestrogen level drops, your blood circulation also slows down; this is a key factor in skin ageing because blood is the nourisher and also the rubbish collector of the body. But the good news is that today's advanced formulations in skincare are definitely on your side, working with vital elements to defend your skin and help it to look its best.

golden rules in your 50s and beyond

■ **The key word in your 50s and beyond is moisture.** Don't just stick with an all-purpose moisturiser. Instead, layer several products designed to do different jobs, to really boost your skin's natural moisture levels.

■ **It's time to rethink your make-up.** Steer clear of too much powder, which has a tendency to settle into wrinkles and exaggerate them. Your natural colouring is probably undergoing a change – paler skin or lighter coloured, greying hair means it is time to establish a colour code which is right for you and create a whole new look.

■ **Regular exercise and a sensible diet** are still the most effective beauty regime. As well as keeping your figure fit and lean, exercise increases blood circulation, which helps give you younger-looking skin.

'it's never too late to protect your skin from further sun damage. Skin maintains its ability to repair itself well into old age, and even those in their 70s and 80s can benefit from using a daily sunscreen.'

Paolo Giacomoni, Head of Research, Clinique

can you really turn back the clock?

You can if you stop what you're doing! There's little doubt that increasingly active lifestyles and environmental factors are having a dramatic effect on the skin. If you're aware of the dangers, you can start protecting your skin now.

the way we live today

Think about it. More than two holidays in the sun each year means extra UV exposure, and then there's the frequent flying which subjects skin to the stress of dehydration. Longer working hours, eating on the run, copious cups of coffee, sugary snacks – coupled with the stress and pace of life – all overload our bodies with toxins that ultimately leave us and our skin dry, dull and pretty lifeless.

Homes and offices now put skin under permanent assault through over-exposure to central heating and air-conditioning which quickly dehydrate the skin, leaving it dry and super-sensitive. Then you go outside. Whatever the weather, warm sunshine or icy cold winds, exposure to UVA rays 365 days of the year further dehydrates your skin and causes free radical damage deep down, which in turn leads to premature skin ageing. And then there's atmospheric pollution – smoke and traffic fumes. Had enough?

what to do

Daily skincare is all about protection and prevention. Repeated exposure to the environment you live in literally strips away the 'glue' which cements skin cells together, keeps your skin's natural barrier to the elements intact and guards against moisture loss. Here are some ways to defend your skin:

■ **Wear a SPF15 sunscreen every day,** whether it's cloudy or sunny.

■ **Increase your intake of evening primrose oil** which contains gamma-linolenic acid (GLA), an essential fatty acid that helps to strengthen skin cells and boost the moisture content from within.

■ **Eat your daily dose of antioxidants,** which help protect our bodies from degeneration: put red, green and yellow fruit and vegetables, such as tomatoes, oranges, spinach, carrots and grapes, on your shopping list.

■ **Wear foundation.** It acts as a great sunblock, because the tiny powder particles are light reflecting and are made from the same material – zinc oxide or titanium dioxide – as most commercial sunblock products.

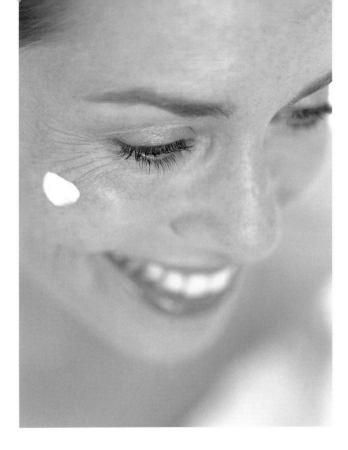

■ **Cut down on caffeine** Caffeine inhibits the absorption of vitamins and minerals. It takes at least a week to wean yourself off coffee. Try drinking herbal teas instead.

■ **Don't eat if you're stressed** It blocks digestion and inhibits the absorption of essential nutrients. Take the time to eat properly and chew slowly, and drink more water. The more you can keep within your skin the better. It helps to flush out toxins from the system, cleansing the body from the inside out.

make lifestyle changes now

■ **Stop smoking or at the very least cut back** It is not only a major health risk, but has been linked directly to premature lines and wrinkles around the eyes and lips. Smoke also restricts oxygen and nutrient supply to skin cells and depletes vitamin C, which is essential for the natural healthy production of collagen in the skin.

■ **Limit your sun exposure** Protect your skin from harmful UV rays. These generate free radicals that speed up the ageing process, so skin sags and bags in much the same way as an apple rots and metal rusts!

■ **Drink less alcohol** Red wine in moderation can benefit your health (the grapes contain powerful antioxidants) but always finishing the bottle won't. Alcohol is sugar, it's also dehydrating and dilates blood capillaries.

■ **Change your diet** The World Health Organisation suggests eating a minimum of 500g (1lb) of fruit and veg a day (that's five apple-size portions). Half the foods you eat should be fresh fruits and raw vegetables, which are rich in antioxidants. To maintain the nutritional content of food, steam, poach, bake or stir-fry.

'about 80 per cent of sun damage during a person's lifetime comes from "incidental exposure" – that is, while out walking, shopping, gardening. Only 20 per cent actually comes from "intentional exposure" to the sun, such as going to the beach. So we need to protect skin all year round.'

Paolo Giacomoni, Head of Research, Clinique

eat yourself younger

'You are what you eat'. We've all heard it countless times before and we probably associate it just with our body image. But how good your skin looks on the outside now, and in the future, really is governed by what goes inside.

working from the inside

'Outward beauty problems are caused by inner problems,' says leading US nutritionist and author, Dr Ann Louise Gittleman. Skin, like hair and nails, can provide a clear indication to the state of your health, and is often the first place to show deficiencies in essential vitamins, minerals, protein and enzymes. 'Dry and dull skin or skin that is too oily or too dry; hair that is lacklustre, thinning or falling out; and nails that are splitting and break easily, are all clues to dietary imbalances,' says Gittleman.

The body is permanently changing and repairing itself and these natural processes depend directly on the quality and quantity of the food we eat. 'Diet is directly linked to skin health,' says Gittleman. 'The popularity of the high-carbohydrate, fat-free diets of the past 15 years has spelled disaster for skin beauty. Blemish-free, glowing skin requires not only a wide variety of nutrients from whole foods rich in protein, vitamins A, C, B complex, zinc, amino acids and essential fatty acids (EFAs), but also needs optimum liver and intestinal function.

'Remember that the skin, like the liver and the gastro-intestinal tract, is an organ of detoxification. If the liver and intestines are overloaded with excess waste – from pesticides, chemicals, heavy metals, solvents, drugs, alcohol, stimulants such as coffee and tea, and processed high sugar foods – 'toxins will inevitably exit through the skin in the form of cysts, bumps, pimples and rashes,' says Gittleman.

Sugar, too, is a hidden enemy. Gittleman has spent the last couple of years focusing on the dramatic effect that excess sugar in our diet has on the ageing process. 'We are a processed generation. It's only recently that we've all wised up to the fact that processed sugar is hidden in everything that hasn't just been picked.'

skin goodies

A healthy diet is essential for healthy skin, so bump up your vitamin C to boost collagen production. Beta-carotene is converted into vitamin A which is essential for cell renewal. Vitamin E, a great antioxidant, helps to control and normalise skin, while vitamin B complex helps to repair. EFAs are vital for keeping your skin soft, smooth and radiant; and the essential fatty acid GLA, found in evening primrose oil, is miraculous for overcoming dryness.

skin baddies

Cut down on: margarine, a hydrogenated fat that blocks the body's ability to use the skin beautifying EFAs; fried foods, which have a clogging effect on the skin's pores; and white flour products (including rice, bread and pasta). Also avoid sugar, which feeds undesirable bacteria and interferes with absorption of skin-enhancing minerals such as zinc, magnesium and calcium; and fruit juice, which feeds yeast that can show up as blotchy, sensitive skin.

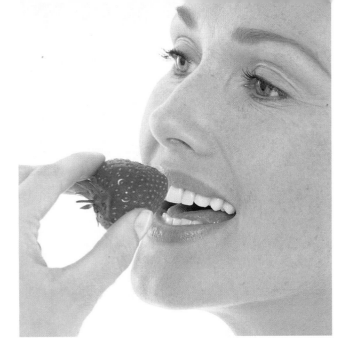

help for acne

Contrary to popular belief, acne is not just a teenage problem but can occur at any time in life, even well into middle age. 'Diet can help to control acne, which can start in your 40s as easily as it can in your teens,' says Gittleman. 'I suggest that any acne sufferers remove all sugar from their diet, including pasta and bread. Try to eat a protein and zinc-rich diet – with organic beef, free-range eggs and lots of zinc-rich pumpkin seeds – that is also high in colourful veggies (green, yellow, orange and red), and fresh salads with a drizzle of olive oil. In addition, for clearing the skin I recommend additional zinc (25–40mg). Cut out copper from the diet as much as you can because copper (found in chocolate, shellfish, and nuts and seeds with the exception of almonds and pumpkin) competes with bioflavonoids: powerful natural antioxidants that help to protect the body and skin from free radical damage and help to boost skin suppleness. Check your vitamin and mineral supplementation. Include a GLA source daily from evening primrose oil and boost your vitamin E levels to help prevent scarring.'

Feed your face

The foods that you put into your body can make a real difference to how your skin looks. These are the top 10 foods for making skin look younger:

- **Avocado** High in the polyunsaturated fat which is crucial to skin softness, and helps boost metabolism.
- **Carrots** are high in beta carotene for well-protected, softer skin.
- **Green vegetables** High in beta carotene, an important anti-ageing, antioxidant vitamin found in carotenoid foods (usually red and green foods such as apricots, carrots, peppers, sweet potatoes and leafy vegetables).
- **Lemon** A good palate and liver cleanser, which also thins the blood. Add a slice of lemon to a cup or glass of hot water.
- **Nuts** Unsalted, unroasted nuts (except peanuts) are high in EFAs to keep skin soft and radiant.
- **Oily fish** (salmon, herring, mackerel) Loaded with EFAs which keep skin plump and dewy.
- **Kiwi** contains five times as much vitamin C, which boosts collagen production in skin, as an orange.
- **Sesame seeds** High in B vitamins, zinc and potassium that support tissues and muscles.
- **Spinach** Rich in iron, it's good for rosy cheeks and gives hair more body.
- **Yoghurt** Promotes gastro-intestinal health and absorption of B vitamins, crucial for skin health.

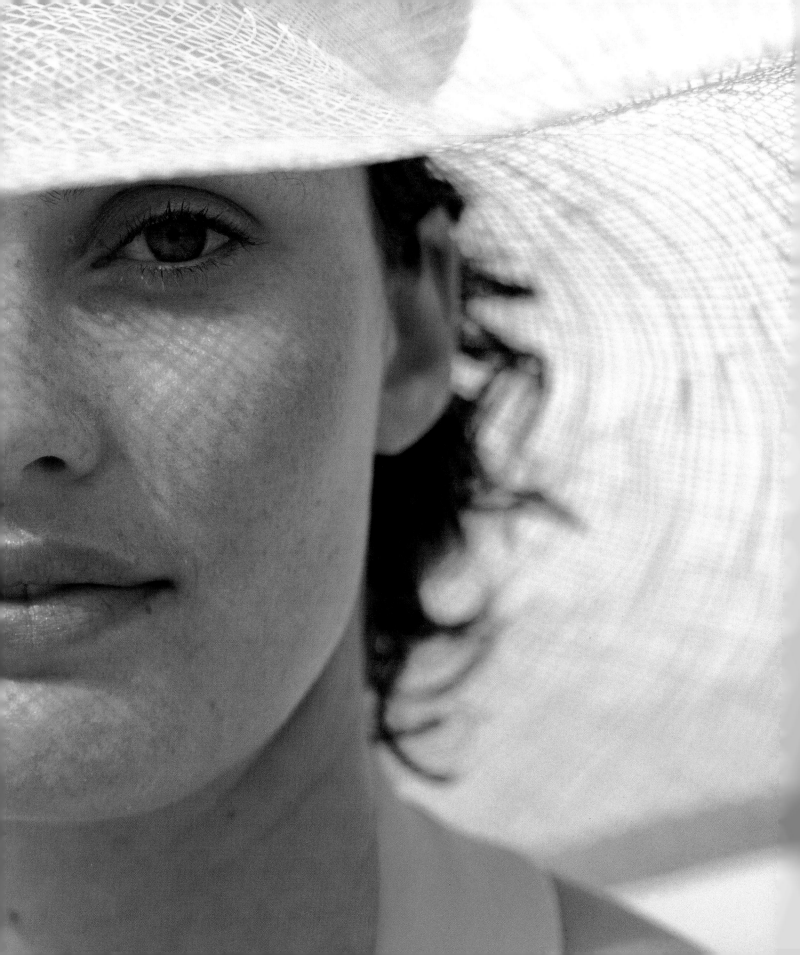

daily skin requirements

why it matters

'Radiant' and 'glowing' are terms we use when someone looks well, but often we're just describing their skin. Follow your daily skincare routine and you will notice a new vitality.

prevention and protection

Daily skincare should be all about prevention and protection, because once the damage has been done, nothing short of surgery will turn back the clock. One blessing is that the skin's natural oils are already there to act as a barrier to stop it from drying out. And although daily abuse from the environment can put this natural protection out of balance, leaving skin dehydrated, your average daily moisturiser can help. Virtually every new face cream is now packed with ingredients designed to help correct this imbalance by naturally supplementing your skin's moisture levels and reinforcing the skin's barrier function to preserve those levels.

Your skin is possibly the most accurate barometer of your well-being, your lifestyle and your age. Young skin is resilient and can withstand all the late nights and general neglect that go with the territory, but mature skin can be unforgiving. It is often quick to mark even brief moments of distress through lack of sleep, exercise, two weeks in the sun, and even experimentation with skincare products that may be too aggressive for fine delicate skin types.

gently does it

Recent controversy over the long-term safety of alpha hydroxy acids (AHAs) – one of the most prolific ingredients of the 1990s – raises concern about how much is too much for your skin. AHAs are used in high concentrations as a drug in many anti-ageing facial peels and in lower concentrations in cosmetic creams, where they exfoliate the top surface layer of skin cells by stimulating the natural cell renewal cycle which slows down with age.

So you get brighter looking skin, fast. However, many skincare experts now believe that some are too aggressive and can actually age the skin as a result. The reason is that mature skin is thinner than young skin and if you thin fine skin even more with exfoliators, you make it more vulnerable and sensitive to UV and other ageing factors. So once again, the key with all skin care is to protect. Make sure you finish your daily regime with a protective moisturiser. Anyone with a mature skin using AHAs, retinols and enzyme activating creams or even a manual exfoliator, should use a daily SPF of 15 or more.

skincare sense

■ **Alpha hydroxy acids (AHAs)** loosen dead skin so that it sheds to reveal a fresher, smoother complexion. Research shows that AHAs can also help your skin retain more moisture and speed up cell renewal. An AHA product can't make skin more taut or get rid of wrinkles, but it can make skin look clearer and more radiant instantly. Some AHAs have been known to trigger skin problems in those with fair or sensitive skin. Citric, glycolic, lactic and malic acids are all examples of AHAs.

■ **Antioxidants** are mostly vitamins – beta-carotene (the precursor of vitamin A), C and E, plus zinc, and a few plants such as green tea and ginkgo biloba (see below). Including them in your diet or taking them as supplements gives the best natural protection from the ageing effects of free radical damage. Antioxidants are often used in skincare and suncare products to provide additional environmental protection.

■ **Enzymes** are natural proteins and currently the hottest thing in skincare technology. Skin naturally contains 'good' and 'bad' enzymes. By harnessing beneficial enzymes and stopping the production of harmful ones, in theory skin becomes better able to protect itself.

■ **Lycopene** is an antioxidant, and is believed to be an exceptionally powerful free-radical scavenger. It is found in tomatoes, pink grapefruit, red grapes and watermelon. A deficiency in lycopene is now associated with skin conditions such as acne and dermatitis.

■ **Retinol** (or retinyls) is the collective term for vitamin A derivatives. They are believed to work in a similar way to Retin-A (the renowned acne treatment from the United States – called Retinova in the UK – which was found to help reduce wrinkles, though it makes skin extremely sun sensitive), only without the irritation. Retinols have been found to help reduce the appearance of age spots and fine lines, and smooth the skin's surface. However, their long-term effectiveness is still unknown.

■ **Echinacea** is infamous for boosting the immune system, has anti-inflammatory properties, and helps to stimulate cellular repair.

■ **Ginkgo biloba** has powerful antioxidant properties. Studies also show that ginkgo leaves help to strengthen the capillary walls, have a moisturising effect, are anti-inflammatory and stimulate the micro-circulation.

■ **Green tea** is another powerful antioxidant, helping to inhibit the release of free radicals in the skin that cause premature ageing. Recent research has shown that green tea alone can reduce the amount of sunburn cells produced under UV light by up to 67 per cent.

■ **St John's Wort** (hypericum) is recognised as an effective natural remedy for mild depression and stress, and also contains huge amounts of skin-regenerating essentials such as flavonoids and tannins.

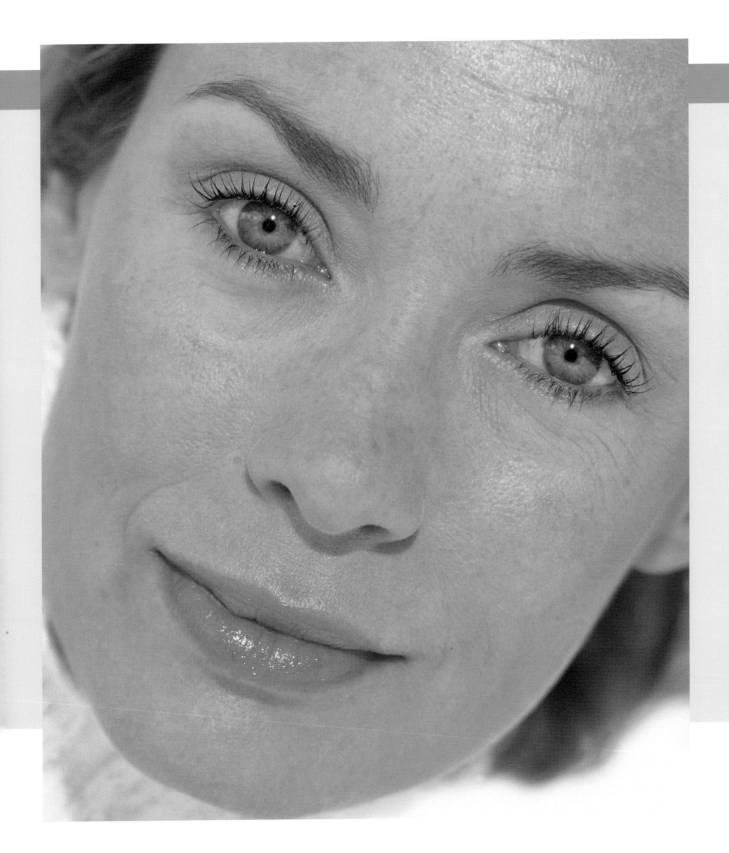

cleansing

Many famous beauties attribute their great skin to a daily cleansing ritual of soap and water. While there are now many equally effective yet gentle cleansers available, finding the right one for your skin will keep it looking its best.

the first step

Cleansing is more than simply keeping your skin fresh and clean. Skincare experts now say it's the first vital step in your skincare regime, helping to prepare mature skin for any additional treatment. However, gentleness is paramount. If a cleanser is too harsh or inappropriate for your skin, it will make it more sensitive and susceptible to irritation. As a rule, always choose a cleanser that won't 'scrub' the skin.

who they're for

Everyone needs to clean their skin from daily dirt and grime. For dry skin, it's better to avoid wash-off cleansers and stick to creams and milks which are wiped away with tissue or cotton wool. Clever new formulas that encapsulate humectants (which attract moisture to the skin) and emollients (which help skin retain moisture) boost your skin's moisture levels even while cleansing.

Oily skins tend to prefer the squeaky clean sensation that goes with rinse-off cleansers, and rarely tolerate a feeling of oily residue, but there's a tendency to be over-zealous, stripping the skin with harsh products that encourage more oil production. Many beauty therapists believe that the best way to cleanse oily skin is to leave moisturiser off the T-zone for a while.

If you have combination skin, the correct cleanser should address both concerns, helping to cleanse as well as balance moisture levels.

If your skin is acne-prone (it doesn't always disappear in your teens), go gentler still on the cleanser and the scrubbing. Acne is believed to be an inflammatory response and strong cleansers and exfoliators can irritate the problem. Look for a very mild cleanser with an anti-bacterial agent.

If you have sensitive skin, it's worth seeking out specific sensitive skin ranges that minimise potential skin irritants, and include many soothing botanical extracts.

how often?

When you wake up, look before you lather. If there's no shininess and your face feels dry, apply a hydrating facial toner and moisturise immediately. If, however, your face is shiny when you wake up, the chances are that it's dirty (since dirt and dust adhere to surface oils) so use a cleanser that suits your skin type. Removing the day's dirt should be a two-step process: facial cleansing and make-up removal. That's because the average cleanser can't cut through the waxes, oils and pigments in make-up to get to the dirt and debris that has built up over the course of the day.

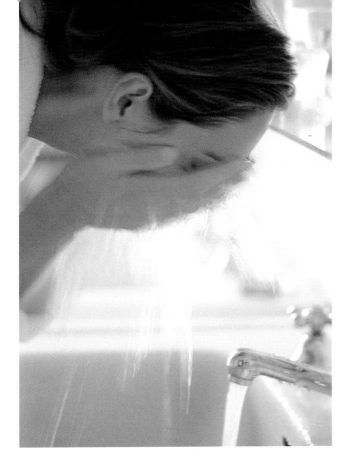

which cleanser is best?

Soap is still a popular choice with those who like the fresh, tingling sensation of washing with water. Soap is certainly an effective cleanser, but when mixed with water it leaves a residue on the skin that can't be easily rinsed away. It is this residue that gives skin that familiar dry, taut feeling after washing with soap. Rinse-off, soap-free cleansers, on the other hand, are carefully pH balanced to match the pH levels of the skin and, more importantly, do not leave any residue on the skin after use. Alternatively, you can choose between a creamy cleanser and a foaming cleanser, both of which are available in such wide ranges that you will easily be able to find one to suit your skin and your lifestyle. Creams are loved by those with very dry, mature skin and often seem a gentle option for delicate skin.

how to cleanse

For dry and sensitive skin, tissue-off types work best and the more emollients (moisturising ingredients), the better. For combination skin, try a creamy rinse-off type; for oily you'll need rinse-off lotions or gels. Whichever type you choose, apply it with the fingertips and massage thoroughly on to your face, around eyes and over the neck using circular movements. The more you massage, the better. Rinse well with fresh water or tissue it off.

to remove eye make-up

If you wear a lot of eye make-up (especially waterproof mascara) or your facial cleanser stings, an eye make-up remover will do the job quickly and easily. Soak a cotton pad with the remover, place it over the whole eye, press on and leave for a few seconds before wiping in a downwards movement. If you prefer an oily remover, it's worth following with a sweep of regular make-up remover because oil from the waterproof formula can cause tears and puffiness if left on overnight. Finish off by wiping beneath the eyes with a cotton bud or cotton wool ball moistened with water.

Daily tips

■ Avoid rinsing with very hot water, it only encourages broken capillaries.

■ Thirty splashes of clean water boosts the skin's circulation and removes any last traces of cleanser.

■ Always use a separate eye make-up remover, especially if you wear contact lenses or waterproof mascara.

moisturising

Every day skin loses a little natural moisture, helped along by changes in season, central heating, air conditioning and extreme temperatures. Daily moisturising can prevent unnecessary moisture loss and preserve youthful skin.

why moisturise?

Daytime skin beauty is all about nourishment: feeding and replenishing your skin with the precious oils and water it needs to stay soft and youthful. Natural oils in your skin act as a barrier to stop it from drying out, but when under attack (from dehydration, central heating, air-conditioning, UV damage and pollution), it goes out of balance. Not enough oil and skin quickly loses moisture, becoming dry, flaky, thinner and less supple.

who they're for

If you're in your late 20s, 30s or early 40s, you will want to invest in the future of your skin, although you are probably less concerned with skin sagging at this stage. Look for a cream with high daily UV protection and anti-ageing vitamins (antioxidants): these are the key ingredients to protect skin from the daily adverse effects of sun pollution, wind and dehydration.

Dry, mature skin benefits from a rich textured cream that gives long-lasting moisturisation. Apply four dots to freshly cleansed skin, on the forehead, cheeks and neck, then gently massage in with your fingers, avoiding the eye area. Oily and combination skins still need moisture to plump up skin cells, but are better suited to a lighter for-

mulation. Choose a light fluid with all the moisturising and technological benefits of a cream.

Tinted moisturiser gives skin a sheer hint of luminous colour and helps even out skin tone, while offering all the vitamin skincare benefits of a moisturiser. These can be used instead of make-up on top of your moisturiser. Apply to the skin using your fingertips and blend from the centre of the face outwards. If you're over 40, or if your skin has been subject to a great deal of sun damage, look for a richer moisturising cream that contains more advanced technological ingredients such as retinol and AHAs.

how often?

Be wary of moisture overload. Experts believe that too much moisturiser makes the skin sag, especially around the eyes, and encourages blocked pores. Beauty therapist Janet Filderman always suggests leaving off moisturiser along the nose, especially if you suffer from blocked, open pores. Bear in mind that if your foundation has added moisturisers you can usually get away with using a lighter lotion underneath. It is important to make sure your moisturiser contains a sunscreen, unless you use a separate UV block.

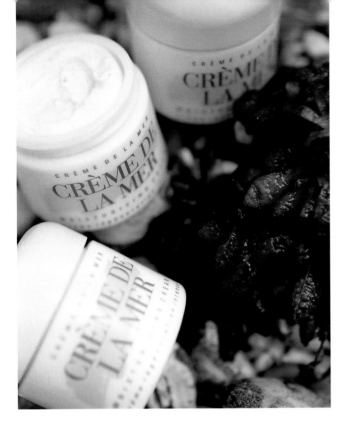

Which is best?

Every moisturiser now seems to contain state-of-the-art, anti-ageing ingredients, but its basic function still remains the same: to act as a barrier and thereby help to keep as much moisture in the skin as possible. All you have to decide is what you really want and need from a daily moisturiser.

■ **Anti-ageing cream** Designed to give dry, mature skin that everyday nourishment, protection and care it needs for ageless beauty and well-being. The latest contain skin refining vitamins A, C and E that help to reinforce the skin's natural barrier function, plus protective UV filters and antioxidants such as green tea and ginkgo biloba.

■ **Oil free moisturiser** The ideal choice for oily skins since they often need moisture, but never oil, in a cream.

■ **Night cream** A good moisturiser can be used around the clock. But if your day cream contains a SPF, you may want to avoid using unnecessary sun filters on your skin. Skin needs beauty sleep to repair, regenerate and rest. According to skincare experts,

skin cells renew themselves faster while you sleep, so this is the perfect time to allow your skin the benefit of a richer cream. However, some experts believe that skin should be left well alone at night, allowing impurities to seep naturally to the surface while you sleep. If you use a night cream and your skin looks oily and congested in the morning, you probably don't need it. If in doubt, leave it off for a few days and see if your skin improves.

■ **Eye cream** Many moisturisers, except those with AHAs or those that are particularly rich and oily, can be used around the eyes. However the skin here is very fragile, which is why specific eye treatment products are lighter and are developed with this in mind.

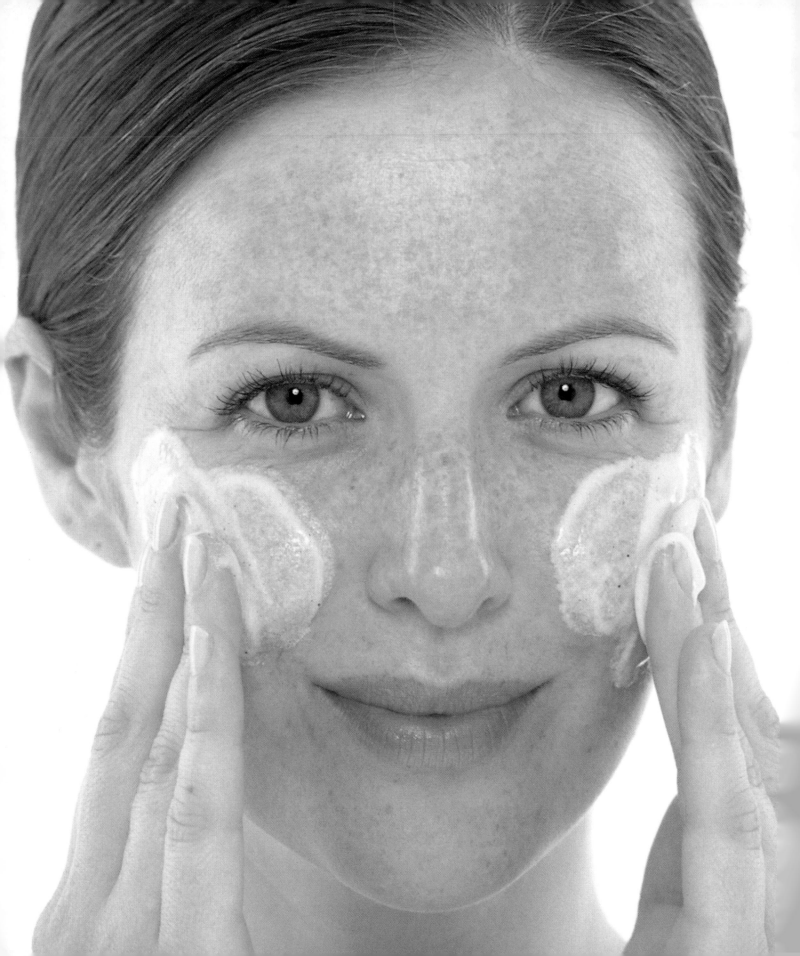

specialist
skin care

On top of your basic skincare regime, take time out to give your skin some special treatment. Face masks pep up all skin types, while exfoliators give tired skin a new radiance.

who masks are for

Most skins will benefit from the regular use of a mask. Skincare experts now believe in the power of layering products on top of each other. The theory – and sometimes even the evidence – is that this way they enhance the action of other products, so your skin gets precisely what it needs at any given time. After all, few skins are oily or dry all over. You get patchy zones of dehydration with oily skin, or dry skin with an oily T-zone: by layering, your skin takes what it needs. So how do you choose? Look carefully at your face and decide upon the main condition of your skin – be it oily or dry – then on a secondary condition, say flaky forehead or dehydrated cheeks, and choose the second mask based on this.

how often?

Beauty experts say that oily skins should use face masks more often and dry skins less, but it's often the other way round. Most masks stimulate skin so it ultimately produces more oil, while dry skin has dead skin cells on the surface that need to be shifted regularly to help normalise the skin's natural renewal process. Therefore oily skins should limit their use, while dry skins can use them at least once a week.

which type?

Oilier skins, which are more prone to blocked pores from excess sebum and dirt, should use traditional clay-based masks (including earth, tar and seaweed extracts) which help to absorb excess oils and impurities, and cleanse pores deep down. If blackheads and congestion are the problem, peel-off masks, which work a bit like exfoliators, are better still. These help to eliminate surface dead skin cells that make your complexion look dull and dirty, making them great for dry and oily skin alike.

skin that feels dry

This could be due to dryness which naturally occurs when skin is quite thin (either from ageing, or simply fair skin types) and unable to retain sufficient moisture. Or dehydration is often caused by air-conditioning, central heating, drinking too much alcohol or coffee, and not drinking enough water. And remember, even oily skin can be dehydrated, because it's water that's in short supply, not oil. Moisturising and revitalising masks come in thick creamy emollients and generally include superior moisturising ingredients such as hyaluronic acid, along with ingredients to stimulate circulation in the skin. They rarely dry on the skin and are used more to plump, soften and iron out signs of ageing and tiredness. Many contain flower, herbal extracts and plant oils to improve the skin's appearance.

tired looking skin

Quickie emergency wake-up masks that refresh definitely rate as a necessity after a late night. Some plump up to counteract dehydration, a few exfoliate too, but most contain menthol, camphor and other cooling, astringent ingredients to boost the circulation, make skin feel tingly and give it a healthy glow. They provide an excellent skin pep any time you need it, especially after a long day or before a party, but other than that do little to deeply cleanse or condition the skin. Don't overdo these: some radiance masks may have a drying effect on more sensitive skins when used too frequently, which can be irritating to skin.

exfoliators

The theory behind exfoliation is that dead cells on the surface of the skin make the complexion look dull and lifeless. Removing them also helps to speed up a sluggish natural cell renewal cycle, that naturally slows down with age. According to Amanda Birch, beauty therapist at Michaeljohn's Ragdale Clinic in London, exfoliation is the key to brighter, fresher looking skin because it removes dull-looking dead cells from the skin's surface to expose younger, fresher skin beneath, and encourages better cellular renewal. Sue Harmsworth of skincare company ESPA agrees. 'Exfoliation is as imperative for the face as it is for the body, to help boost the skin's natural renewal cycle and for better absorption of moisturiser and other treatment products.

who they're for

Everyone can benefit from exfoliation. Done regularly, it can help skin creams to penetrate faster and more effectively, making skin instantly appear softer and smoother. However, there is growing concern about just how much is too much. While young skin (15–35 years) is thick, supple and resilient, older skin (over 35 years) is thinner and ultimately more porous and susceptible to external damage. And while it helps to make skin look brighter and clearer at any age by sloughing off these dead skin cells, experts now say you don't want to make fine skin thinner still or it may even accelerate environmental ageing. Only by understanding your own skin will you know what you can or cannot get away with. Exfoliation is extremely beneficial, but it's never good to do anything to excess.

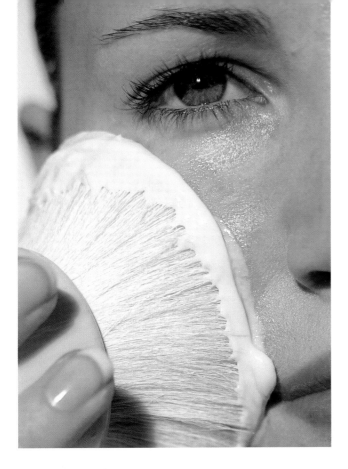

how often?

This is constantly under debate, and no two skin specialists ever agree on how often it should be done. However, in skincare less is more and exfoliation is quite an aggressive action, so oily skins should exfoliate once a week, dry skins should exfoliate once every two weeks, and if you have sensitive skin take it easy and only exfoliate perhaps once a month if your skin needs it. Exfoliation should be concentrated around those parts of the face that are most prone to oiliness, open pores and blackheads – such as the nose, chin and forehead – which is why oilier skins benefit the most from this type of treatment. Never use it around the eyes and always apply moisturiser immediately afterwards.

which one?

You can exfoliate your skin manually, using a grainy scrub, a buffing cloth, or a chemical exfoliant such as an AHA cream or an enzyme cream. Grainy scrubs contain tiny particles which, when massaged into the skin, help to lift out dirt and impurities and rub off the dead skin cells that otherwise cling to the surface of the skin, then they are rinsed off. The best to choose are perfectly rounded spherical beads that are less likely to scratch the surface of the skin, unlike walnut and apricot grains cut from the kernel, which often have sharp particles that may damage the skin's surface. A muslin face cloth is considered a much gentler way to buff the skin. However, a soft cloth or flannel will do the job just as effectively.

Exfoliating or peeling creams or lotions often contain enzymes or AHAs (alpha-hydroxy acids). Enzyme exfoliators generally contain naturally occurring enzymes, such as papain from papaya, or bromelian, the enzyme found in pineapple. When left on the skin for a few minutes, these gentle but effective enzymes work by dissolving the dead skin cells, leaving skin brighter and smoother. AHA creams work by loosening the top layers of dead skin so that they shed to reveal a fresher, smoother complexion. Research shows that AHAs can also help your skin reinforce its own protective barrier function as well as its ability to renew itself. However, AHAs have also been known to trigger skin problems in some women, especially those with fair, delicate or sensitive skin.

anti-ageing facials

Having a facial isn't just about having layers of creams and masks to plump up and soften your skin, though that's certainly part of the allure. It's also taking time out for yourself – a pampering experience that goes way beyond skin deep.

talk to your therapist

Ideally every facial should have a mini-consultation beforehand. Make sure you tell the therapist if you are pregnant, have a medical condition (epilepsy and a pace maker are clear contra-indications for CACI and other non-surgical facelift treatments) or are using a skin treatment cream such as Retinova (or Retin-A)

Remember, it is your time and your money. Always say if you are not happy about something, whether it's the temperature of the room, you're not keen on the music they're playing, you're uncomfortable, or there's a part of the facial that you don't like. Here are eight of the best for mature skins:

■ **Academie lifting & firming treatment with vitamin C** Particularly suitable for oily skins, because of its astringent action, this facial helps skin to recover its firmness and tone, and a temporary lifting effect is usually observed immediately afterwards. The skin is first cleansed and exfoliated before a concentrate of pure vitamin C is applied, along with seaweed pads. These are then massaged into skin. Then comes a face mask, which is left on for 10 minutes before being wiped off with damp sponges. This is followed by the application of a protective day cream to finish the treatment. As a result, skin looks firmer and the complexion brighter.

■ **CACI (Computer Aided Cosmetology Instrument)** One of the first and still considered the most effective 'non-surgical face-lifts'. It uses a low frequency microcurrent to help stimulate the facial muscles, thereby improving muscle tone and skin elasticity, albeit temporarily. Great as a one-off treatment for a special occasion or as a course of treatments to give your skin a boost, devotees often remark on the 'lifted' effect it gives to skin.

■ **Clarins Paris Method facial** This is one of the most relaxing facials imaginable because it is simply a series of therapeutic massage movements using deliciously scented skincare products. Its unique form of massage (still kept a closely guarded secret) was developed by Jacques Courtin-Clarins, originally a physiotherapist. It involves over 70 highly specialised massage movements, each of which has a very different action on the skin. Some help to decongest a blemished skin, some to detoxify and reduce puffiness, and others to firm and tone or simply to relax. Throughout a Paris Method treatment the only tool the beauty therapist uses is her hands. This means that every type of skin can benefit from the facial, regardless of its condition.

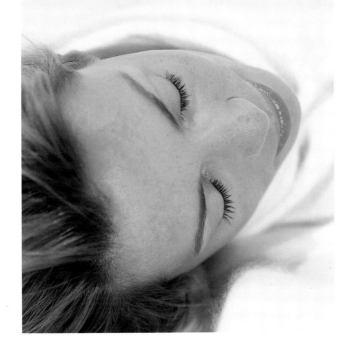

■ **The Dr Hauschka facial treatment** This is more than just a facial, it's a unique two-hour mind and body treatment that aims to re-balance and re-harmonise the skin and body in one. It begins with a sage foot bath to warm and relax you, followed by a foot and leg massage, a hand and arm massage, and a scalp massage, to prepare you for the rest of the facial. Then a hot aromatic lavender compress is applied to your face and you take deep breaths in.

Cleansing is warm, gentle and rhythmical, working down the face to begin the detoxifying processes. The therapist continues working down the face to stimulate the body's lymph system and encourage the skin's natural detoxification processes. Homeopathic ampoules are applied to balance your skin and finally you are treated to a neck and shoulder massage using blended essential oils. At the end your skin, and your whole being, are left feeling calm and soothed from head to toe.

■ **ESPA luxury facial treatment for mature, dry, dehydrated skin** This treatment concentrates on reviving the skin's natural moisture levels and pays particular attention to the delicate eye area. It involves a pressure point massage, lymph drainage and a combination of hydrating, nourishing and replenishing aromatherapy products to leave the face and neck totally revitalised.

■ **Gatineau Filmomasque facial** This moisturising treatment is both incredibly relaxing and superbly rehydrating for the skin. It consists of a cleanse, tone and marvellous facial massage, followed by a mask that sets like rubber. After the mask has been pulled off, a daytime moisturiser is applied.

■ **Guinot Hydradermie** (Previously known as Guinot Cathiodermie.) Guinot was the first company to use electrotherapy combined with plant-based skincare products in a salon facial. It is considered to be the ultimate deep cleansing facial, and leaves skin super clean. The face is scrubbed, cleansed and steamed, then tiny metal rollers are massaged over the skin from the neck upwards. This is followed by a face mask, then cleansing takes place once more. It's surprisingly relaxing, and the effects are long-lasting.

■ **Thalgo2 oxygen therapy facial** A richly moisturising facial ideal for dry skin types; skin feels exceptionally soft and supple after treatment. The facial begins with a thorough cleanse of the face and neck followed by exfoliation. Then the skin is sprayed with a fine mist of an exclusive vitamin cocktail, using the Thalgo 'oxygen massager'. This takes about 20 minutes using specific uplifting anti-wrinkle movements on the face and neck. A moisturising O_2 Lustre Mask is then applied as the finishing touch, followed by a daytime moisturiser.

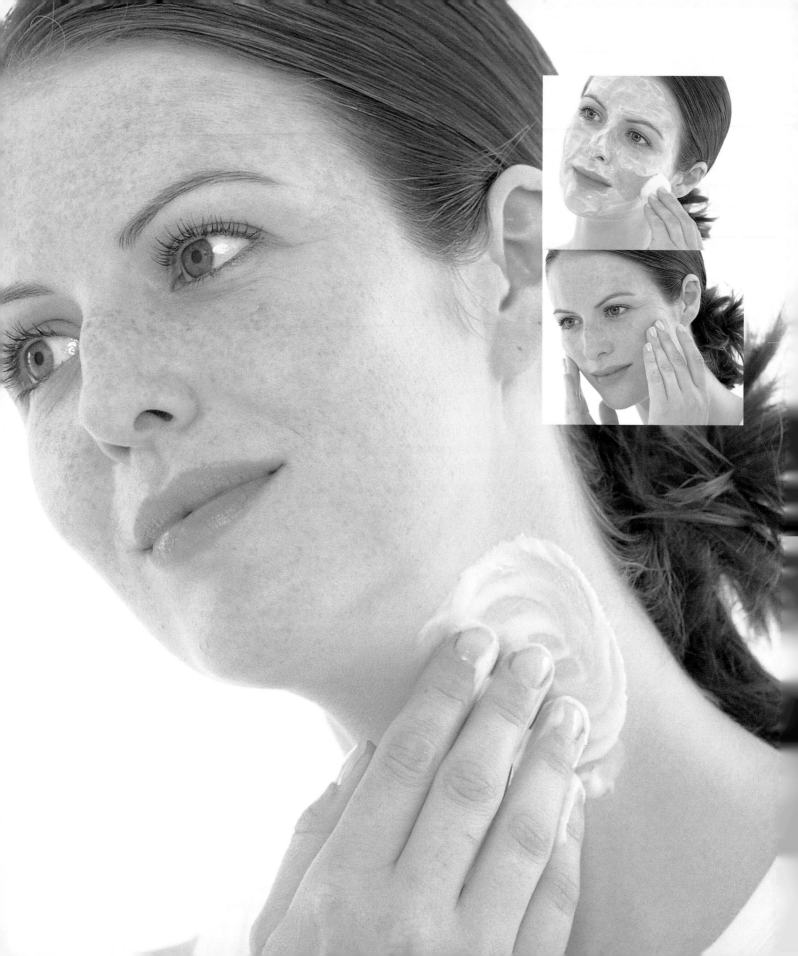

DIY home facial

A home facial once a week for just 15 minutes, on top of your usual daily skincare regime, can make a real difference to your skin and the way you feel.

Cleanse and tone Cleanse your skin with a creamy cleanser, which always feels more pampering than a rinse-off cleanser. Warm it between the palms of your hands, then massage it into your skin with firm, circular movements. Take a clean tissue, make a tiny slit in the middle and place it over your nose, pressing the tissue on to your skin to help it absorb any excess cleanser. Finally wipe off the remaining cream. Use a toner to refresh your skin and help to remove any last traces of cleanser. A facial spritzer is a great pick-me-up for your skin at any time.

Steam and exfoliate If you have normal to oily skin, try a little light steam. Fill a bowl with hot water, then add a few herbs such as lavender, chamomile, basil and rosemary. Tilt your face over the bowl with a towel draped over and steam for between two and five minutes, depending on how sensitive your skin is. Now gently exfoliate your skin to remove any dead skin cells. Choose a gentle face scrub, with smooth micro beads that won't scratch. Rinse your face and neck thoroughly with warm water, then spritz again.

Apply a face mask Choose either a deep-cleansing, clay-based mask for oilier skins or a moisturising cream mask if your skin feels dry. Lie back for five to 10 minutes, depending on the mask,and place a couple of chilled chamomile tea bags on closed lids to soothe them as you rest. Remove the face mask, then spritz skin again to help remove any last traces of the mask and apply a little aromatherapy facial oil. Look for one containing rose essential oil, which is especially nurturing to dry, mature skins.

Massage your skin Now massage your skin using the oil. You can brighten the complexion and help detoxify the system by massaging pressure points across the face and eye area to improve the lymphatic drainage around the face. Placing your four fingers on both eyebrows, press slowly, then release. Repeat this process three times. Then move your fingers to the lower socket area (just under the eyes) and, again, with light and slow pressure, repeat three times. Sweep the fingertips up to the centre of your forehead and press along outwards towards the temples on either side. Continue to press along the hairline, past the cheekbones, pinching the earlobes, and pressing along the jawline until your fingertips finally meet at the chin. Try to incorporate this basic pressure massage as part of your regular skincare regime, even when you are just smoothing in a little face cream. Finally, blot off any excess oil with a clean tissue, and apply your usual moisturiser or night cream, depending on the time of day.

eyes

As we're all too aware, the skin around the delicate eye area is the first place to show wrinkles. It loses moisture more quickly than anywhere else on the body and needs daily care and protection to stay looking youthful.

effects of ageing

Your eyes are one of the first places to show the visible signs of ageing. The skin here is incredibly fine and delicate, and more readily absorbs UV light, the ultimate skin damager. It also has less collagen and elastin to keep it supple, and loses moisture more quickly than anywhere else on the body. A total of 22 muscles constantly crinkle this vulnerable area when you blink, squint and crease your eyes in reaction to sun, wind, smoke and cold, and computer screens.

importance of protection

It's said that our eyes are the 'windows of our soul', and they mirror what's going on inside the body, too. Lack of sleep, exercise and fresh air, stress and many illnesses are revealed in your eyes. The rules for eye health are pretty basic: they should be protected from strain, glare, dust and dirt. Just like the rest of the body, they need relaxation at frequent intervals. Sun exposure accounts for 80 per cent of wrinkles, so they need extra protection from UV light.

Diet is important, too: a poorly balanced diet will result in dull, tired eyes. The most nutritious foods for eyes contain vitamin A: citrus fruits, apricots, green leafy vegetables, carrots, turnips, egg yolk, butter and cheese. To keep your eyes clear and sparkling, drink more water, avoid excessive amounts of alcohol, too many late nights, too much sun and don't smoke.

how to care for your eyes

Sensitive eyes respond quickly to any fingertip pressure along the acupressure points. When they feel particularly tired, sit with your elbows on a table in front of you, and lightly interlock your fingers, placing both thumbs between your brows. Allow your head to rest on your thumbs, lightly bearing the pressure. Hold for a count of five, then repeat in six steps along the brow. Finish by sitting up and gently pressing with your middle fingers along the delicate area underneath each eye. This technique is also great for removing puffiness.

'Palming' is another gentle pressure massage used to stop facial puffiness. With fingers pointing up towards the top of your head, gently press the heels of your hands on to the tops of the cheekbones. Rest palms gently on your eyelids so that you feel the heat they generate. And a popular tip from beauty therapists is to keep eye gel in the fridge so it feels more refreshing when patted over tender, tired or puffy eyelids.

Eye remedies

■ **For sore, tired eyes,** soak and chill two chamomile tea bags (used ones are fine), lie down and place on closed lids for 10 minutes. If your eyes feel irritated, too, try eyebright. Either buy teabags and soak them before applying to closed eyelids, or buy the liquid and add to a bottle of water and drink throughout the day. Eyebright is particularly helpful for minor cases of conjunctivitis, sore, red eyes due to dust or grit, styes and eye strain.

■ **To wake up sleepy eyes,** place two cotton wool balls that have been soaked in ice cold milk over your eyes for five minutes.

■ **For puffy eyes,** sleep with an extra pillow to help prevent fluids from 'pooling' around the eyes.

■ **If you have crow's feet,** regularly apply eye gel or cream and wear sunglasses with UV100 protection.

■ **Apply cream to the eye area** You don't need to use a specific eye product, but you're less likely to get watery or puffy eyes from cream slipping into the eye if you do. Apply cream as far as your laughter lines reach – screw up your eyes to see exactly where they are. And don't drag or pull this delicate skin when you are cleansing and moisturising your eyes: simply tap gels or creams gently into the surrounding area.

■ **If your eye cream always ends up in your eyes** regardless, dot a tiny amount on the browbone only. Here it will melt into the skin and be absorbed all round the eye during the night.

■ **The most effective way to remove mascara** is to soak a cotton wool ball in eye make-up remover lotion, hold against the lashes and lightly press into them, then stroke downwards without tugging. Rubbing is hard on the eyes, and cleanser may leak into your eye.

■ **Wear sunglasses on your eyes,** not on your head! It's the best defence you have against wrinkles

■ **Have a regular check-up** every six months with an optician, especially if you already wear glasses or contact lenses. Try to reduce the wearing time of your contact lenses, and buy a couple of stylish glasses frames that suit your personality and dress sense as well as your face.

■ **Improve your light** Tired, watery eyes may indicate eye strain. Always have lights brighter than you think you need them while using computers, reading, sewing or doing other close-up work. Or try using a reading lamp, directing it onto whatever you're doing, but do take shadows into account.

neck

We all appreciate an elegant, swan-like neck. However, before we even begin to realise what's been going on, skin here becomes dry, lined and crepey. Prevention is better than cure, so start protecting this area now.

effects of ageing

Perhaps even more revealing than your eyes or your hands, your neck and décolleté can readily give your age away. Skin here is thinner and drier than the face, with fewer naturally protective sebaceous glands to guard against moisture loss, so it's prone to crepiness. Soaps, detergents and perfume all dehydrate and sensitise the neck to other irritations such as polo-neck jumpers, scarves and extreme weather conditions.

importance of protection

This is an area where prevention is much better than cure. Once the skin on this bony area of the body is lined, it is extremely hard to turn back the clock. You should aim to protect this frequently exposed zone from daily environmental exposure.

how to care for the neck

Carry your regular skincare regime beyond the jawline and on to your neck and chest. Cleanse your neck and décolleté gently, using your regular cleanser or facial wash. Every two weeks, use a gentle exfoliator to smooth and soften the skin and allow creams to penetrate better. Moisturise night and day with a lotion or serum, both of which absorb quickly into the skin and are less likely to leave a mark on your clothes. Specialist neck lotions contain many of today's popular high-tech ingredients, such as retinol, AHAs and enzymes, and you may find that regularly applying a moisturiser to this previously neglected zone will help to nourish the skin and make a noticeable difference.

neck remedies

■ **Exercise your neck.** Every time you apply neck cream: lightly stroke upwards from your chest to your jawline, 15 times, using the backs of your hands. Then lightly slap under your chin with the back of one hand, 20 times very fast. Finally, using one hand, place the fingers on one side of your neck and the thumb on the other side, and make firm but gentle circular movements up and down your throat six times, then repeat with the other hand.

■ **Daily use of a sunscreen** whenever your neck is exposed is vital. Use either a daily moisturiser with built-in SPF15, or a separate sun protection lotion.

■ **Wear jewellery.** Diamanté, pearls – the bigger the better – will draw attention away from your neck while people gaze at the jewels and wonder if they're real.

■ **Wrap it up.** Whether it's a long scarf or a high-necked jumper, once wrinkles are there you may feel more confident if they are kept where they can't be seen.

hands

Always on show, your hands and nails say a lot about you. Smooth, soft hands and buffed and polished nails reflect good grooming. Left unprotected and unkempt, they say you just don't care.

effects of ageing

Rarely protected as much as the skin on your face, hands are always on show and permanently exposed to the elements. As well as dryness and wrinkles, hands most commonly develop age spots and raised veins, mostly due to UV exposure.

importance of protection

UV light is your hands' worst enemy. As well loss of elasticity and suppleness, it causes age spots. These are due to an uneven clumping of the skin pigment melanin and their appearance can, to a certain extent, be lessened. Certain ingredients now used in hand creams incorporate mulberry root extract or hydroquinone, which work by breaking down the skin's pigmentation just below the surface.

Your fingertips are valuable indications of your physical well-being. Common nail problems include white spots: once thought to be caused by excess calcium or zinc in the body, these are actually the result of a bump or from pushing the cuticle back too harshly. Ridges, like wrinkles around the eyes, are usually due to ageing. Brittleness is associated with ageing, too. Fragile nails can indicate dietary deficiencies, particularly a lack of protein, while spoon nails – when the nail curves upwards in the shape of a spoon – may be hereditary or reflect anaemia, poor circulation or, occasionally, coronary disease.

how to care for hands

Moisturise liberally with a rich hand cream every time you wash your hands. Wear an SPF15 sunscreen daily; always wear protective gloves in winter, and when doing housework or gardening.

hand and nail remedies

■ **If your hands are very dry,** massage in plenty of hand cream before going to bed and wear a pair of cotton gloves over the top.

■ **To boost circulation in your hands,** try this exercise used by pianists. Clench both hands into a tight fist, then open them out again really quickly, stretching the fingers out as far as they'll go. Hold for a count of two. Repeat 10 times.

■ **If you have short, square or narrow nails,** select a nail varnish colour close to your skin tone and you won't draw attention to them.

■ **If you have ridged or uneven nails,** use a frosted or pearl shade (or a ridge filler under your polish).

■ **If your nails are wide,** leave a narrow strip on either side of the nails unpolished to make them appear narrower.

■ **If you have long, thin nails,** leave the very base of the half moon of the nail unpolished to shorten them.

■ **If you have chipped polish,** carefully dab in the polish using several thin layers in the same colour, then apply two coats over the entire nail.

lips

Next to eyes, your lips are the most expressive part of your face, and a barometer of how you live your life. They can tell a stranger whether you're happy or sad and are first to show the signs of dehydration and fatigue.

effects of ageing

The skin on our lips is made up of an entirely different structure to our facial skin. It is thinner and finer even than the delicate skin around our eyes, and lacks several of the body's protective substances, including an effective lipidic barrier, which helps to keep moisture within the skin and makes it soft and plump. As we get older, our lips naturally get thinner as they lose some of their fat. And gradually, the fragile skin around the lips becomes prone to fine lines. So after eyes, our lips are among the most vulnerable areas in the fight against ageing.

importance of protection

Lips need extra protection from the drying effects of the environment: sun, wind, pollution, central heating and air-conditioning. They lose moisture regularly (licking your lips often makes them even drier) and they contain no sebaceous glands to keep them oily and supple. That's why it is important to protect them daily. UV light causes up to 80 per cent of skin ageing, and since the lips have no natural protection in the form of melanin, it is important to apply a sunscreen, or a lip balm with at least SPF15.

Your lips are also a prime site for cold sores (encouraged by sun exposure) and some skin cancers, and many dermatologists believe that using a high SPF protection can significantly reduce the risks. Lipstick offers some daily UV protection: the more intense the colour, the better the protection. Typically, however, fashionable summer shades are often more sheer, so you'll need an additional SPF balm underneath.

how to care for lips

To keep lips looking younger for longer, keep them regularly hydrated with a daily dose of lip balm or lip salve, and re-apply regularly throughout the day. These products are made up of a fatty substance such as beeswax or carnuba wax which seals the lips and acts as an invisible barrier to keep moisture in. The surrounding skin should be kept moisturised, too, to prevent lines from appearing. Use a moisturiser with crucial skin-saving vitamins A, C and E and a sunscreen to protect skin from premature ageing. This is especially important if you are a smoker.

lip remedies

■ **If you suffer from chapped, scuffed lips,** take a tip from professional make-up artists. Apply lip balm regularly. If there is a loose piece of skin, don't pull at it. Instead, liberally apply Vaseline petroleum jelly and use an old, clean toothbrush to rub gently away at the skin. It's the best way to exfoliate your lips.

■ **If you are a smoker,** you are more than likely to end up with deep, tell-tale lines around your mouth. This is caused by the smoke itself as it swirls up around your face, eyes and lips, releasing skin-ageing free radicals which break down the essential collagen and elastin that keep skin looking young and supple. If you can't stop smoking, then at least try to up your intake of the antioxidant vitamins A, C and E.

■ **For a DIY conditioning lip mask,** give your lips a coat of vitamin E oil. Mix 5ml of this oil with one drop of rose oil. It gives lips an instant natural shine without colour and helps to condition and protect their sensitive skin. Apply at night and never under lipstick – oils make colour slide off in seconds which is why that healthy salad at lunchtime has eradicated your carefully applied lip line.

■ **If you have fine lines around your mouth,** apply your usual moisturiser over your lips as part of your daily skincare regime. Lip primers have conditioning formulas to provide a no-bleed base for lipstick, and protect your lips from becoming dehydrated. Use a lip pencil to accentuate your natural lip line and to hold colour in place through the day.

■ **If you find your usual lipstick is drying throughout the day,** try using a lip primer beforehand. This will help to condition your lips but, unlike lip balm, it gives the colour something to cling to, so your lipstick should stay in place a little longer.

■ **Say your vowels – a, e, i, o, u.** Repeat them as if speaking in slow motion 20 times a day. This is a good facial exercise and can be a great pick-me-up when you're feeling tired.

■ **Finally, get a little laughter into your life.** It brings a light to your eyes and a smile to everyone's lips, especially yours. And let's face it, better to have lines which turn upwards after a lifetime of laughter than those which turn down from a lifetime of sorrow.

skincare solutions

■ **If you have a shiny T-zone,** try leaving moisturiser off the area for a few days (many contain mineral oil which tends to clog the pores). Then, to keep it in check throughout the day, try a T-zone control gel (Lancôme and No7 do one) that contains powder particles to absorb oil.

■ **If you suffer from puffy eyes,** this could be caused by lying flat at night: it's often a result of fluid retention, and looks worse in the morning. The most refreshing eye remedy is a couple of cotton wool balls dipped in ice-cold milk then applied to the eyes. Leave for five minutes then rinse with fresh water and pat dry.

■ **If you have dry, cracked lips,** protect them with lip balm, preferably one with SPF15. Re-apply the balm as often as you can remember throughout the day, rather than waiting for them to get dry. Resist licking your lips: this only makes them drier.

■ **If you regularly suffer from blackheads around the hairline and cheeks,** use only cosmetics which are 'non-comedogenic' and won't cause comedones (blackheads). If the blackheads are around your nose and chin – an area that often produces more oil naturally, anyway – your pores may be getting blocked too easily. Try steaming and exfoliating once a week.

■ **If your skin feels very dry and lacking in vitality,** increase your water intake. Aim to drink a 1.5 litre bottle of mineral water throughout the day. Any more, and you may place additional pressure on your kidneys.

■ **If your skin feels tight after cleansing,** you may be using the wrong type of cleanser. Soap binds with water to form insoluble deposits on the skin which make it feel extra dry and sometimes itchy. Choose a soap-free cleanser instead.

■ **If you have tiny red thread veins,** avoid using very hot water on your skin, and protect your skin in extreme temperatures. Wear a moisturiser daily, and an SPF 15 to prevent further damage.

■ **If you regularly suffer from spots, blemishes or acne,** it might be worth looking at your diet. Many skin problems are aggravated by certain foods such as citrus fruits and dairy foods. Eliminating these from your diet for a couple of weeks could make a significant difference.

■ **If you frequently have skin problems** around certain areas of the face, such as the hairline, chin and jawline, it could be due to your own bad habits! Avoid touching your skin throughout the day. Try to break daily habits such as toying with a fringe or hair at the sides, holding your face in your hands, and rubbing your chin or nose with your fingers.

■ **If you suffer from an allergic reaction** on your face or around the eyes, bear in mind that it may be due to something on your hands (including ingredients used in nail polishes). If you rub your eyes after touching something else, the irritation will be more likely to appear pronounced around the sensitive eye area than on your hands.

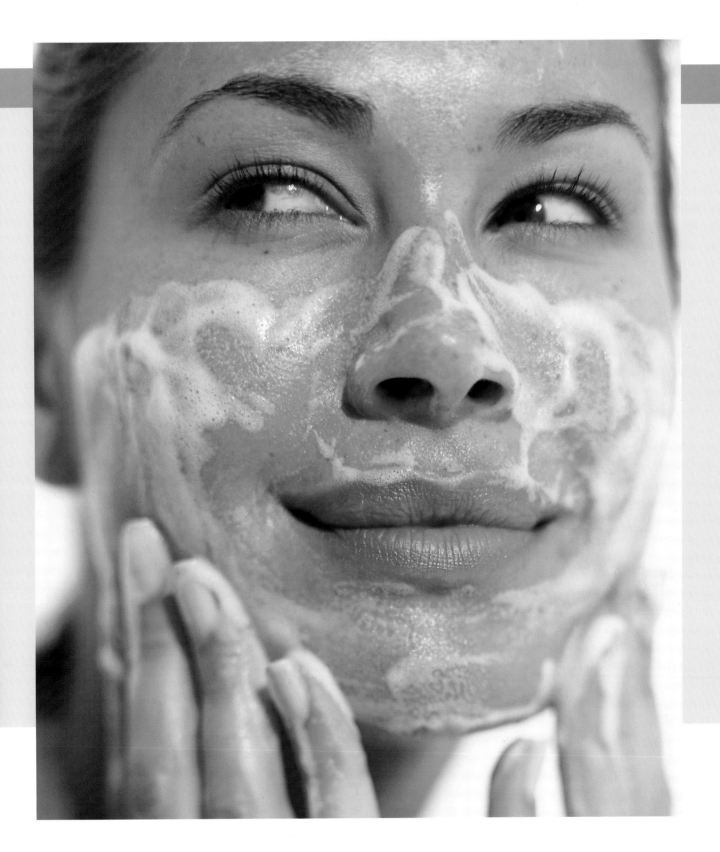

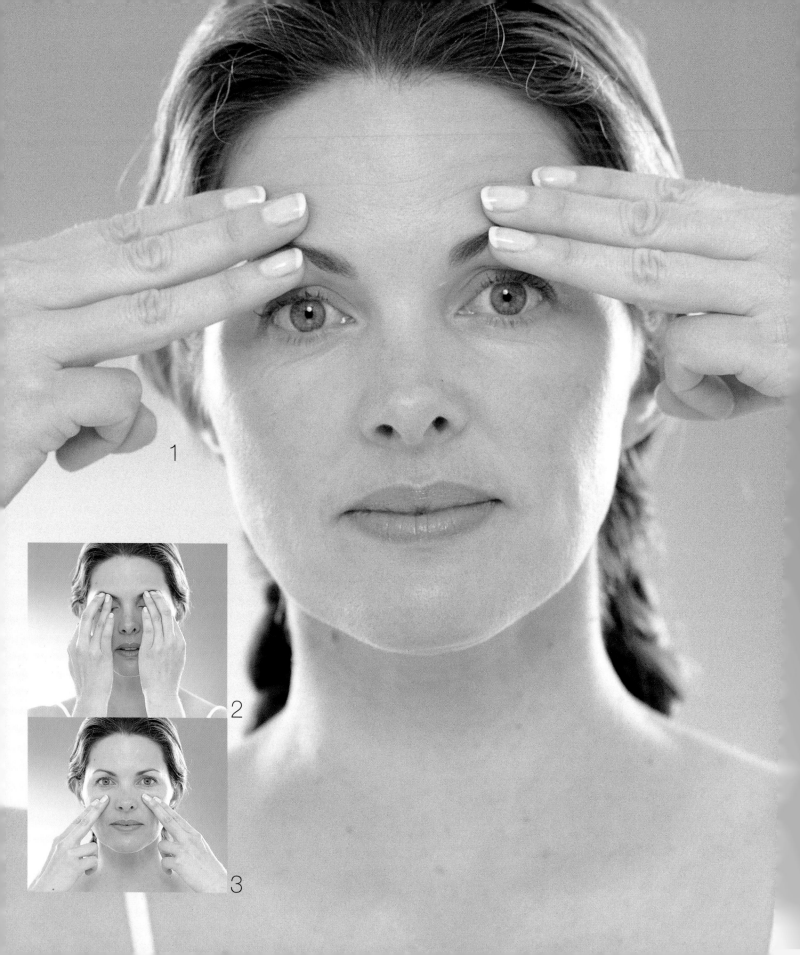

anti-ageing facial massage

Amanda Birch, beauty therapist at London's Michaeljohn Ragdale Clinic, offers this quick pressure point massage, to relieve tension and give a more youthful look to your face.

1 To smooth frown lines and lateral lines on the forehead Start at the bridge of the nose and apply pressure with the middle fingers. Then glide up to the edge of the inner eyebrow, press and glide over the brow to the outer edge, press and glide over to the temples, press and release.

2 To lift eyebrows With middle fingers together, place all three fingers of each hand under each eyebrow; press and release. Glide up to the brows, press and release. Then do two more movements up the forehead towards the hairline.

3 To relieve puffy eyes and sinuses Using the index and middle fingers only, start at the bridge of the nose and work outwards across the upper cheek towards the temple in four movements. Then repeat across, and finally under the cheekbone.

All about facial massage

While a facial massage may sound like the kind of indulgence most of us would rarely make time for in the daily scheme of things, skincare experts believe that it can help to boost circulation, and improve skin tone and firmness. 'The ideal time to massage your skin is while you're cleansing.' says Amanda Birch. 'A good cleanser should simply sit on your skin, unlike a moisturiser which is absorbed, so it makes it easier for your fingers to glide over the skin.' Or if you prefer massaging in the evening when you have more time, Amanda suggests mixing a blend of 3ml of wheatgerm oil with one drop of rose essential oil for an aromatic facial oil.

To massage: Using your middle fingers (index, middle and ring fingers), unless otherwise stated, each movement involves a firm but gentle 'press and release' action with the fingertips on each pressure point, then gliding the fingertips along to the next point shown, and pressing again. Perform on both sides of the face at the same time. Repeat each step three times, daily if possible.

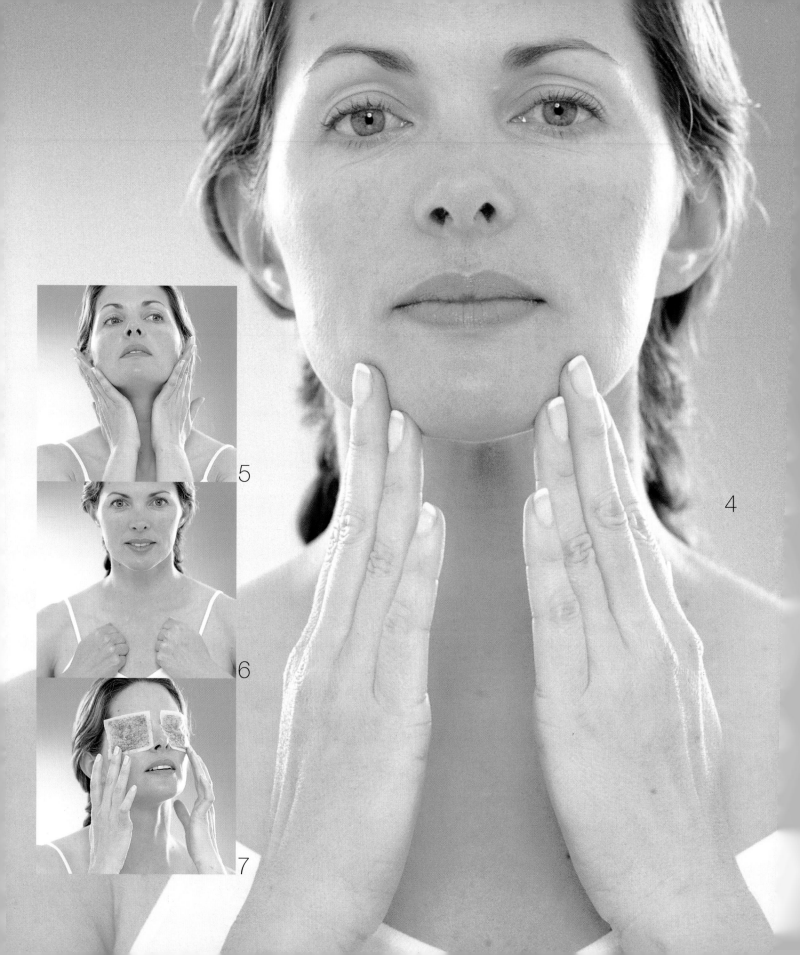

4

5

6

7

4 To boost circulation and brighten the complexion Starting from the centre of the face, massage using tiny, light sweeping upward movements. First start along the browline to the temples, then across the forehead to the temples, then four more down the face, first starting under the eyes, then from the sides of the nose and finally from the chin out towards the ear.

5 To lift the neck Use upward sweeping movements with the fingers and palms from the clavicle bone (should we explain what this is or is it clear from pic) up to the jawline.

6 To stimulate the décolléte Use light and gentle kneading with the knuckles along the décolléte area. Repeat three times.

7 To finish Place a couple of chamomile tea bags that have been soaked in cold water over your eyes and massage the temples for one minute.

Facial exercises

Laughing, talking and shouting on a hourly basis should count as a pretty intensive daily workout in itself. But there are a few specific facial workout routines which are believed to help exercise certain muscle groups that may help to keep your face firm and younger looking for longer. If nothing else, a workout for your facial muscles is also a great way to relieve tension when you're feeling particularly stressed, and after a time it could even help to avoid negative expression lines, such as pursed lips and a down-turned mouth, that come with age.

Try the following exercises first thing in the morning to help you feel more awake and energised. To make the exercises as effective as possible, you need to do each movement as slowly as you can, and imagine that you are working against resistance.

1 With elbows on a table, look straight ahead and place both thumbs under your top lip with the nails resting against your upper teeth and gum. In one slow movement, gently move your upper lip muscles toward your thumbs, hold for a count of five, then slowly release. Repeat 15 times.

2 Keeping your mouth slightly open, smile repeatedly every second, 20 or 30 times. This will strengthen your jaw muscles and prevent the sides of your mouth from turning down.

3 Say your vowels: a, e, i, o, u. As a great pick-me-up when you're feeling tired, repeat your vowels 15–20 times, saying them as slowly as you can, and exaggerating each one as you say it.

your body

it's the only one you've got,

so make the most of it.

Love and appreciate your

body a little more every

day, and take inspiration from

its strength, suppleness

and total uniqueness

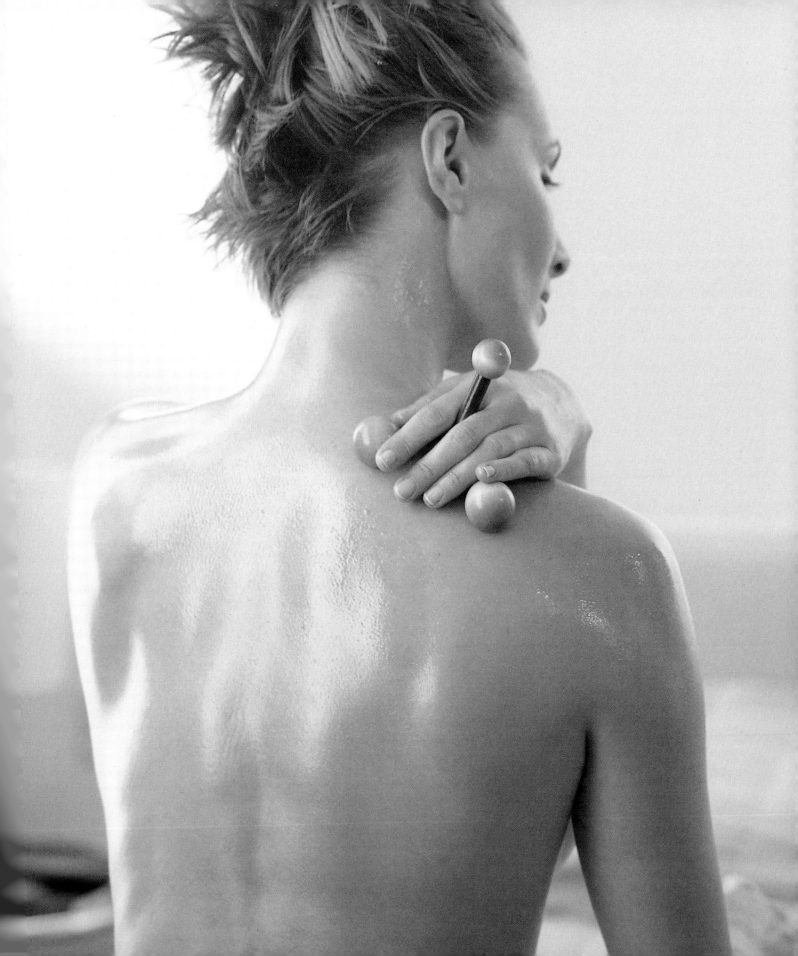

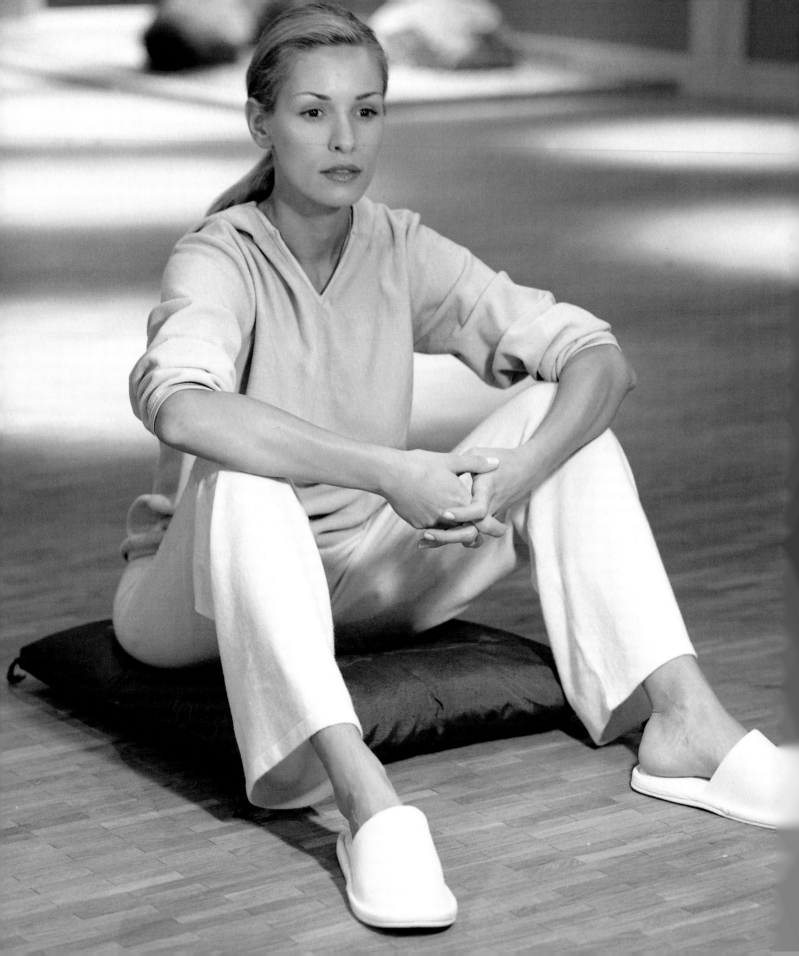

how and why the body ages

what's going on

Hidden under layers of clothing from one season to another, it's easy to forget to look after your body. But, just like your hair and face, your body deserves regular care and attention.

listen to your body

Niggling pains, aching back, or just dull, lifeless hair. Our body constantly sends out signals about our own health and well-being. If you take the time to look and listen, you can actively help to keep your body looking and feeling its best for longer.

It is now estimated that over 80 per cent of visits to the GP are for stress-related complaints, from skin disorders (such as psoriasis and eczema), hair loss and high blood pressure, to depression, heart disease and cancer, which shows that so much of our health – and future well-being – is in our own hands. However, the sad fact is that we continue to neglect ourselves, physically and psychologically.

So now's the time to change lifelong health patterns. Ask yourself how you're feeling, listen to your body and monitor it regularly, so that when things do go out of sync, you will be more aware of your body's reaction to changes and better equipped to deal with them.

how fast is your body ageing?

Are you stressed? At the very least stress can make you feel under pressure, tense and irritable, but at its worst it can lead to the development of a whole range of illnesses, and has been linked to cancer and clinical depression.

reduce stress now

Organise your day and your life, and prioritise tasks properly to make the most efficient use of your time. Become assertive – we're all guilty of it, but learn to say no, so you don't take on too much work. Eating properly is important. Reduce your sugar intake and don't skip meals, but ensure you eat a well-balanced diet to help your body to cope better in the long run. Boost your vitamin levels, especially zinc and vitamin C. Make more time for your partner – sex is a great stress buster. And, however busy you are, make some time for relaxation. Try complementary therapies such as aromatherapy, reflexology and acupuncture.

what's your weight?

Most of us need to lose a pound or two here or there but if you want to check whether your weight really is healthy or not, all you need is a tape measure and a set of scales. Measure your height in metres and weight in kilos. Calculate your body mass index (BMI) by dividing your weight by the square of your height. So if you are 1.6m tall and weigh 60kg, your BMI is 23.4

$$\frac{weight}{square\ of\ height} = BMI \qquad \frac{60}{1.6 \times 1.6} = 23.4\ BMI$$

Ideally you should score between 20 and 25 – anything over 25 is considered overweight, less than 18.5 is underweight, and over 30 is considered obese.

check your posture

Slouching and curling up in front of the television do nothing for your posture and can affect digestion and the function of all your internal organs. According to Pilates exercise expert Alan Herdman, 'Standing up straight gives the illusion of instantly losing 5kgs without doing a thing.'

Check your posture by standing up straight and looking in a mirror. Does your neck jut forwards? Keep it level. Are your shoulders rounded? Scrunch them up to your ears, then relax them down. Does your tummy stick out? Pull it in. Weak tummy muscles are responsible for the majority of back problems.

■ **Avoid carrying a heavy bag on one shoulder;** carry two lighter bags – one in each hand – so that you are balanced. If you have to carry a small child, alternate between hips.

■ **Change the height of your heels.**

■ **If you are working seated at a desk** for long periods of time, ensure that everything is at the right height for you and that you have adequate support for your back.

■ **The Alexander Technique** is a simple system for learning good posture. It prevents slouching and re-educates the way you sit. Osteopathy is the soft-tissue treatment which re-balances the whole body by manipulating the joints.

energy levels

Are you constantly lacking in energy? Do you need more than eight hours' sleep? Are you irritable, having difficulty concentrating, suffering from anxiety, need a cup of coffee to get you going? These are all signs that your health is suffering because your stress levels are high and your energy levels are low. Too much stress has been linked with skin disorders, asthma, PMS and high blood pressure. Cut down on energy sappers such as sugar, alcohol, smoking and stress. Your body loses its reserves of vitamin C, B and zinc when the pressure is on. Boost your intake of vegetables, cereals, nuts and fruit.

Find a method of stress relief that suits you. It might be walking the dog, going for a swim, playing soothing music, having a long, relaxing bath and switching off – or taking up a therapeutic activity such as yoga, t'ai chi, meditation or visualisation. Whatever you choose make it something that you enjoy and that works for you, so you will constantly turn to it in stressful situations.

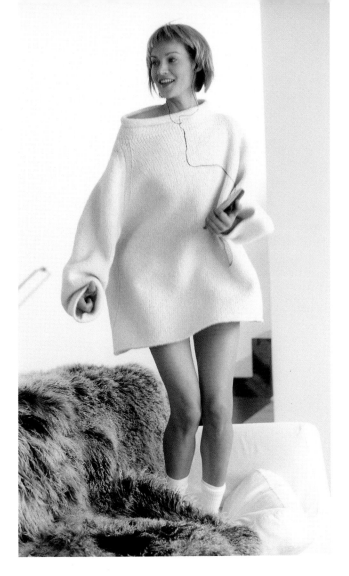

reduce sugar levels

Are you a chocaoholic? Do you constantly feel the need to eat cakes and sweet, sugary foods? It is important to keep sugar levels in check, for not only do they affect weight, but the initial high is quickly followed by tiredness, low self-esteem and irritability. In fact the worst thing you can do is eat something sweet when you feel low as it causes blood sugar levels to rise too quickly, only to fall even more.

Instead, eat a healthy fibre snack such as rice cakes, a banana, crudités (cut up raw vegetables such as carrots and celery into batons), or nuts. Eat small well-balanced meals throughout the day and don't skip on breakfast. It takes about three to four weeks to turn around a sweet tooth, but if you stick to it you will discover new energy levels and handle stress better.

How stressed are you?

Work out your stress rating by ticking the boxes that frequently apply to you.

Physically, do you suffer from:
- fatigue
- frequent headaches
- fainting
- food cravings or loss of appetite
- lack of libido
- restlessness or sleep problems
- tearfulness
- nausea
- skin problems
- excessive perspiration
- feel dependent on alcohol, drugs, cigarettes?

Mentally, do you feel:
- irritable or angry
- depressed or melancholic
- worry about very minor things
- fear failure
- fear disease
- indecisive
- deny problems
- feel isolated
- avoid confrontation?

Fifteen or more ticks indicate a stress level that could seriously damage your health. Talk to your doctor, and discuss your feelings with close family and friends.

can you turn back the clock?

Accepting your body's strengths and weaknesses, and making regular improvements, will ensure that you maintain health and vitality for many years to come. Regular exercise will boost your fitness and help to maintain your weight.

fitness and ageing

There's no denying it, you are the life you lead. Just as many aspects of your lifestyle affect your skin and hair, factors such as stress, poor diet, lack of exercise, insufficient sleep and poor posture all ultimately lead to poor self-image and accelerated ageing from within. Body fitness is crucial to how your body ages. Exercise increases blood flow and volume, strengthens the heart and lungs and lowers your resting heart rate to combat stress – all of which help you to accomplish daily activities with less physical effort and fatigue, so ultimately you really can live longer and look and feel younger if you look after yourself. As you get older your body loses flexibility, so to keep a normal range of movement and maintain quality of life, you need to take regular exercise. By strengthening and improving suppleness, you can prevent your body from becoming stiff and your muscles deteriorating.

increase exercise

If you think your life is too busy to fit in a regular exercise routine, think again. All you need is a basic 20 minutes a day, three times a week, to start getting your body moving. It doesn't have to be 20 minutes of sweaty aerobics; just a brisk walk to buy the daily papers will get you going. Finding a balance that is right for you is the most important thing. The benefits of safe, regular exercise include better digestion and increased strength, stamina and suppleness. Exercise also reduces depression, increases circulation and mental clarity and boosts the immune system.

We all seem to forget that exercise is meant to be a pleasure. Avoid making it another stress or burden that you'll begrudge doing. Do something you enjoy: dancing, roller-blading and trampolining, for example, are fun forms of exercise. Combine that with a swim once a week, a couple of brisk walks and maybe a yoga or Pilates class and you're already on your way to a balanced exercise regime.

use exercise to increase energy

■ **Tune into your body rhythms** Exercise when your energy is at its highest: it'll be easier to make the commitment. Research shows that morning exercisers stick to it more than those who exercise at the end of the day.

■ **Try something new** A change in an established body routine can make a difference to the amount of vitality you feel.

■ **Relax to recharge** While aerobic exercises have proven training effect, yoga, t'ai chi and other mind-body exercises also offer energising effects.

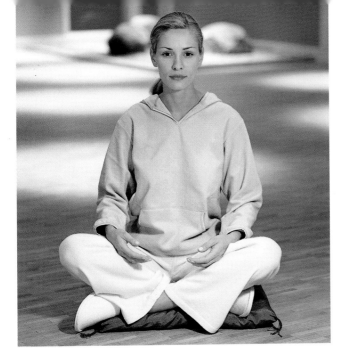

inner cleansing

Skin is a living organ which reflects your inner health. Pollutants such as alcohol, coffee, tea, the chemicals involved in the processing of food, medical drugs and cigarette smoke take their toll on your skin's freshness and clarity.

When overworked and burdened with fatty foods, alcohol or emotional stress, the liver's efficiency is reduced. As a result, toxins accumulate in the blood and can show up on the skin, causing it to look blotchy and blemished. Skin expert Eve Lom recommends a citrus fruit and water fast for two days to give the liver a rest and help stimulate organs (ask a doctor's advice before fasting and never attempt if pregnant). Citrus fruits (limes, grapefruit, lemon, orange) help to fortify the liver and are also rich in vitamin C, one of nature's most potent detoxifiers and antioxidants.

Encourage kidneys to flush away toxins by drinking masses of mineral water, which is free from the chemicals found in ordinary tap water. The easy passage of food through the intestine is vital for the cleansing process, so roughage or fibre, found in the leaves, stalks and roots of vegetables as well as in the skins and seeds of fruit, will help.

Top five energy drainers

It is totally within our power to boost our energy levels simply by the way we live our lives.

■ **Smoking** cuts down oxygen delivery to body tissue and less oxygen means less energy.

■ **Dieting** The amount of calories you take in has a direct effect on your energy level. A low-calorie diet (less than 800 a day) forces your body to draw on muscle tissue for energy, leaving you feeling weak and listless. Too much refined sugar makes our bodies sluggish and our spirits fatigued, although the initial rush of energy we get is often the reason we consume so much of it. Cut it out and see the difference it makes to your energy levels.

■ **Stress** is a mental and physical energy drainer and leaves you with less get-up-and-go.

■ **Alcohol** is both a dehydrator and a sedative. A glass of wine at lunch may leave you feeling fatigued later that afternoon. Drinking in the evening can lead to fragmented, restless sleep, affecting your energy levels the next day.

■ **Exercise** Too much or too little is an energy drain. Balance out your life.

ways to stay young

■ **Increase your activity.** Obesity is more of a problem than ever in the UK with over 50 per cent of us overweight. Long-term effects of obesity include diabetes, heart disease, muscle and joint problems, and back problems. Aim to exercise three times a week for 20 minutes at a time.

■ **Seek the positive in all things.** Until you accept yourself, no amount of healthy eating or exercise will help you look or feel better.

■ **Cut back on alcohol.** Drinking a glass of red wine now and then can actually benefit your health: the grapes contain powerful antioxidants called procyanadins, which protect the body from the inside out. But all things in moderation: no more than seven units a week. (One unit equals one standard glass of wine, 300ml (1/2 pt) beer or a single measure of spirits.)Too much may give you more than a hangover, and in the long term can cause conditions such as stomach problems and high blood pressure.

■ **Increase the amount of coloured fruit and vegetables** in your daily diet. These are full of anti-ageing, health-giving antioxidants which prevent degeneration throughout our entire body. The recommended amount of fruit and vegetables is five 'apple size' portions, which is equivalent to around 500g (1lb) in weight. Wherever possible, eat fruit and vegetables raw or lightly steamed to preserve all their nutrients.

■ **Eating a well balanced diet** will give your body the full range of vitamins and minerals it needs, along with essential proteins, unsaturated fats and carbohydrates, to stay fit and healthy. Reduce your intake of saturated animal fats which are known to increase the risk of heart disease and have been linked to other diseases. The World Health Organisation recommends that fats should comprise a minimum of 15 per cent of your daily calorie intake, and no more than 40 per cent. Nuts (almonds and walnuts) and oily fish (herring, sardines, tuna) are good sources of unsaturated fats and essential fatty acids.

■ **Cut down on caffeine.** Like any stimulant, the effects of caffeine are wide-ranging, including exhaustion, nervousness, irregular breathing, high blood pressure, mood swings, digestive disorders and headaches. Caffeine inhibits the absorption of vitamins and minerals. It takes at least a week to wean yourself off the effects of coffee, but you will feel surprisingly energised. Drink herbal teas and hot water with lemon instead. Or try green tea, a natural source of antioxidants.

■ **Take the time to eat properly.** Chewing your food slowly has been found to help relieve stress and tension.

■ **Drink more water.** As well as flushing potentially harmful toxins from your system, water hydrates the skin and energises the body.

■ **When you're stressed,** the adrenal glands go into hyperdrive. Practise simple deep breathing techniques, meditation or yoga, to induce a state of calm.

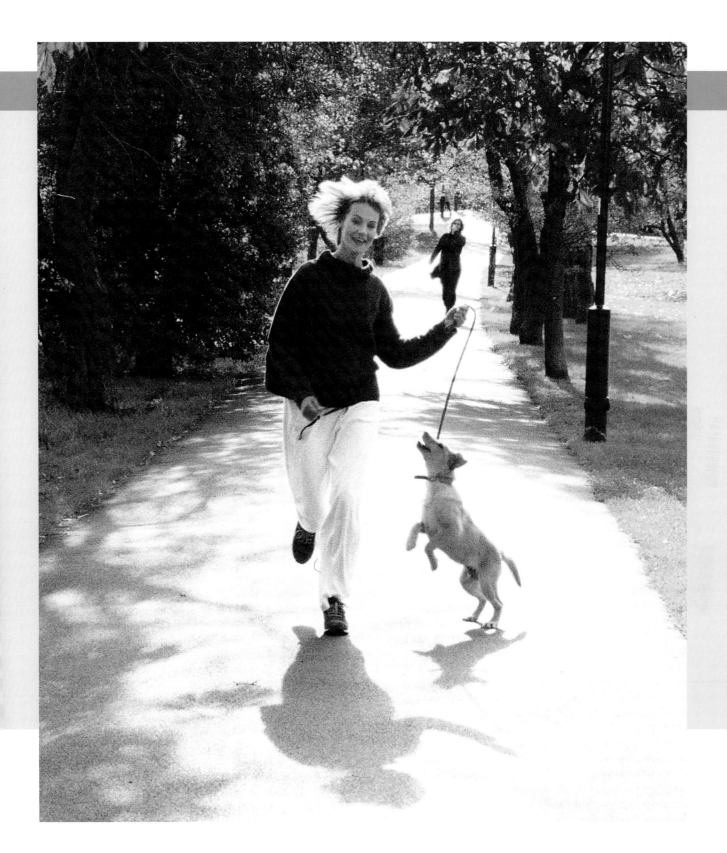

body boosting tips

Easy short cuts to achieve renewed vitality and abundant energy.

■ **Taking a bath is one of the best ways to detox,** says sports and health expert Dr Laz Bannock. 'A shower won't do it. You need to lie submerged for at least 10 minutes to allow the osmotic effect of water to help draw out toxins.' (Skin and body cells perform a re-balancing act, drawing essential water and nutrients in from the bath, and toxins out of the body.)

■ **'Add 1 kg of Epsom salts to your bath'** says Liz Earle, lifestyle author and creator of the Naturally Active Skincare company. 'It will leave you feeling floppy at first, but it's wonderfully restorative, and people never add enough for any real benefit.'

■ **Indulge in a yawn or two:** it's your body's way of getting more oxygen to the brain, increasing mental clarity at the same time.

■ **Drink more water.** You've heard it all before, but water is vital for energy, clear skin and bright eyes. Aim for 1.5 litres taken throughout the day, and not just all at once or you'll overload the kidneys. Dehydration reduces blood volume so you're circulating less oxygen to the body, and will ultimately feel more sluggish.

■ **Give yourself a soothing back massage.** Place two tennis balls in a sock, space them two inches apart and tie a rubber band around the open end. Lie down comfortably on the floor and position the balls on either side of your backbone. Gently roll yourself up and down, concentrating on particularly tense areas.

■ **Start cutting back on sugary snacks now,** and boost your intake of colourful fruit and vegetables in their place. Just knowing that you are making an effort and aiming in the right direction will boost your confidence tenfold.

■ **If you suffer from fluid retention,** increase the amount of mineral water you drink. This will help to flush out toxins within the body which encourage bloating and puffiness.

■ **Focus on the positive.** Think of the features of your body you like, such as a warm smile, long, elegant hands or strong arms.

■ **Deep breathing clears the head** and sets you up for the day, especially when you're under pressure. Try this breathing exercise: sit upright on a chair or the floor, with your hands resting on your tummy. Breathe in fully, count to two, then breathe out for a count of six at the same rate. Be aware of your hands rising and falling. Repeat 12 times.

■ **Remain seated and try this massage technique** to calm the senses and enliven the mind. Firmly press the fleshy part of both ears from the lower lobe upwards. Do this twice, then lightly press your fingertips along the brows, into your temples and along the nape of your neck.

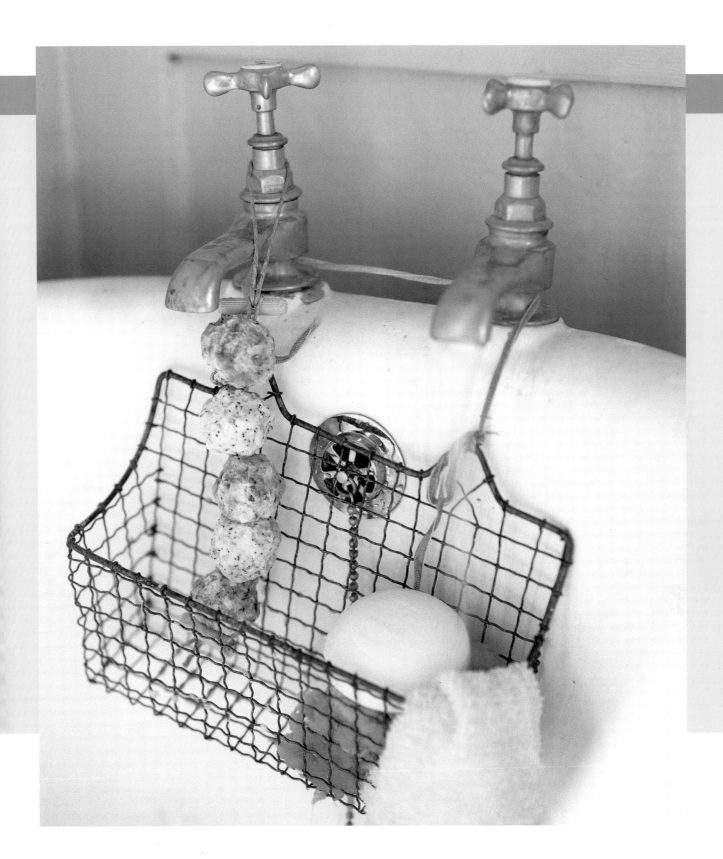

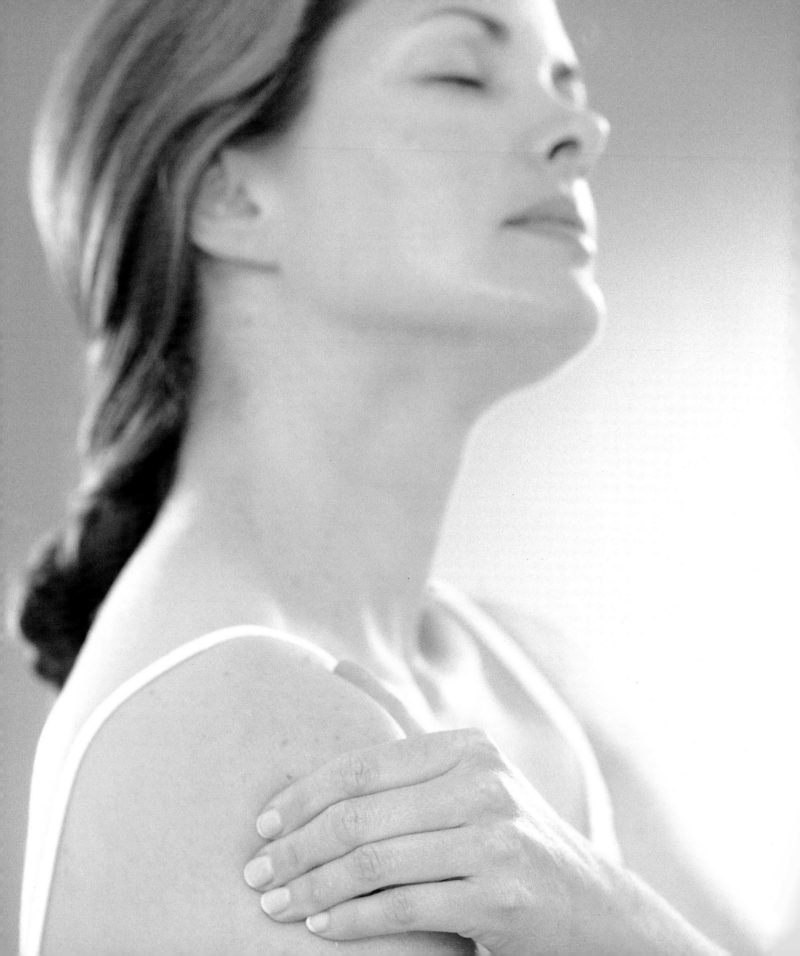

daily body requirements

why it matters

You've got to love your body. The more attention you lavish on it, the better it will look and the more you will appreciate it. How can anyone else love you if you don't love yourself?

beauty from within

The most beautiful people are those whose beauty shines from within, whose character, not bodies, represents how the outside world sees them. So start to love your own body. Follow a healthy lifestyle, go to the gym, have regular massages. Pamper your body and pay it some real attention at last – it's never too late! Ultimately it is all about being happy. When we are happy we are more positive, relaxed and accepting of all things, so life feels in balance. Stress and worry can age our appearance and affect our health, whereas fun and laughter are rejuvenating. Research continues to show how laughter releases the body's own pain relief, which speeds up the healing process.

the value of touch

Touch is an essential part of our well-being and you might consider some established massage techniques. Aromatherapy massage uses fragrant essential oils from a wide variety of flowers, plants and herbs, to relax, revitalise or re-balance your whole being. Shiatsu massage works by applying pressure alone to various energy points along meridians associated with the functions of different organs throughout the body. Reflexology uses massage and finger pressure on the soles of the feet to stimulate specific energy points and help restore energy flow throughout the body. Seek a professional at all times: specific zones around the ankle may be too stimulating during pregnancy. Similar in many ways to Shiatsu, the eastern therapy of acupressure massage uses the fingers to apply pressure and stimulate specific energy points throughout the body.

Swedish massage was developed during the nineteenth century and is a system of strong, sweeping strokes that helps boost circulation and lymphatic drainage. It's great for tired legs and puffy ankles, but some therapists can be too vigorous, so go by word of mouth. Osteopathy uses touch and manipulation of the skeletal system to improve the body's own healing powers and promote a sense of inner calm.

bathing and moisturising

Daily body care goes beyond just getting clean. Simply washing with soap, scrubbing with an exfoliator or massaging in body oil puts you back in touch with your body and the more you make of it, the better you'll feel about yourself.

bathing as therapy

In the UK, we either bathe or shower: rarely do we do both. But, says French beauty therapist Anne Semonin, in order to fully enjoy the experience (and reap all the benefits from the products you use on your body) you should do as the Japanese do and combine the two. 'Use the shower to scrub and clean your skin, and the bath to soak and treat the body and mind with therapeutic additives such as pure essential oils.'

Bathing is undoubtedly more therapeutic than showering. Recent research in the USA found that our first response to 'stress overload' was to retreat into the bathroom. After all, where else can you indulge for 10 minutes, an hour or a whole afternoon and emerge a whole new being? Now that's got to be the best therapy. When the body is immersed in water, nearly 90 per cent of its weight is displaced: you feel lighter, slightly suspended and instantly at ease. Warm water promotes tranquillity too, because it lowers your blood pressure, but any hotter than 30°C and skin will get dehydrated, make you feel floppy (because it raises the body temperature) and may cause broken capillaries.

blissful ways to bathe

Using therapeutic bath additives and body oils you can create the perfect mood at any time of the day: uplifting and energising first thing to help you focus on the day ahead, or restful and relaxing to help you keep calm and reflect, and improve your quality of sleep.

energising morning bath

■ **Start with dry body-brushing** to stimulate your body's lymphatic system, then take a quick shower to get yourself clean before you bathe.

■ **Run a warm bath,** then add two drops of juniper oil and two drops of cypress oil for a herby pick-me-up.

relaxing evening bath

■ **As a haven of pure relaxation,** a soothing, soporific soak is one of the nicest ways to switch off at the end of the day. Set the scene: dim the lights, and light a scented candle.

■ **Add three drops each of neroli, geranium and lavender** essential oils to still bath water, step in and immerse yourself in the fragrant warm water.

rejuvenating bath tips

■ **To soothe away stress and ease tension,** rest your neck and shoulders in the bath with a travel pillow.

■ **As you soak in the bath,** put on a face mask, or place some soothing eye pads over your closed eyelids.

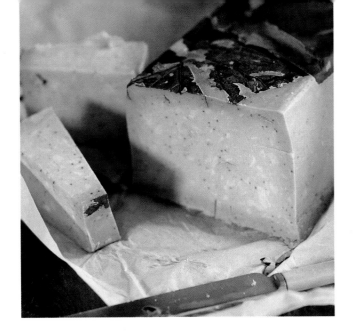
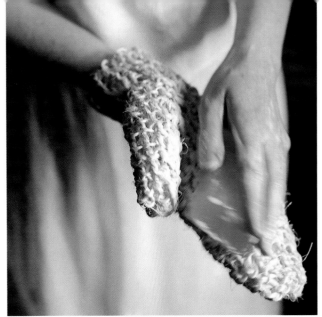

when to moisturise

Whether you bathe or shower, scrub or just soak, always follow with a body moisturiser to help seal moisture in the skin and prevent further dryness caused by the water. Every supermodel's number one tip for gorgeous body skin is to moisturise. Massage in plenty of creams, lotions or oils, whichever you prefer. This will keep skin gleaming and, even if you've been neglectful, can make a big difference in just a few days.

'It is always advisable after exfoliation, or daily bathing, to replenish the natural oils which are lost not only through washing, but through pollution, air conditioning and the environment generally,' says Susan Harmsworth of ESPA. 'A hydrating body lotion should be applied onto damp skin on a daily basis.'

which type to use?

You can now find the same high tech skincare ingredients in your body cream as in your face cream.

■ **If you like cream** You can get away with using a heavier cream on your body than you can on your face, and the body is less sensitive to skin-smoothing AHAs and retinols. Gently but firmly massage creams into the skin in a clockwise circular movement to help stimulate your circulation and digestion.

■ **If you like lotion** These are absorbed more quickly, making them perfect for use after a morning bath, or when showering in the gym.

■ **If you like oil** You can use any oil – even those you'd use for cooking, such as olive, sunflower, hazelnut and almond oil – but specialised body oils tend to be much more refined so they absorb more easily. Try mixing your own: just 10ml of oil mixed with six drops of your favourite essential oil. Apply preferably at night so the oils can be left to absorb and have more benefit, and you don't risk leaving an oily stain on your clothes.

■ **If you like a perfumed body moisturiser** Virtually every perfume now comes with its own scented bath and body range. However. while you may love the smell of your favourite fragrance, it is worth remembering that moisturisers, whether cream, lotion or oil, sit on the skin, so the fragrance may smell slightly different as it isn't interacting with your skin so much. And don't overdo it: you can't apply fragranced body moisturisers quite so liberally. If you want to use them, you could use an all-over moisturiser first, then just use the perfumed one in selected areas.

toning

It isn't always our actual size that bothers us, but our lack of firmness and tone. There's little doubt that a body that looks fit, firm and smooth and relatively 'dimple-free' is preferable to one that wobbles as you walk.

improve skin texture

Greyish, blotchy, bumpy skin and cellulite, which are mainly attributed to sluggish circulation and poor lymphatic drainage, can still be improved with a variety of treatments. And often, just the action of massaging in a cream to the hip and thigh area can improve the texture of your skin, making it feel softer, even if it doesn't look any smoother.

brush your body

Dry skin-brushing is an intense form of body exfoliation. As well as smoothing skin and boosting circulation, it is an invaluable part of detoxification, helping to stimulate lymphatic drainage and eliminate up to 30 per cent of the body's waste. It should be done before showering, on dry skin with a soft-bristled brush. It involves brushing the skin, using a bristle brush, in firm upward sweeping movements towards the heart. Do this each morning before bathing, while the skin is dry. Brush the entire body, paying particular attention to problem areas such as the thighs and backs of arms. 'I do it every day, and it takes just two minutes,' says beauty therapist Amanda Birch 'It is one of the most effective treatments, helping to boost dull skin on the body, treat cellulite and relieve puffy ankles.' Start at the feet and work up the legs, then the hands to the shoulders.

toning treatments

Ionithermie is a salon treatment for cellulite. It combines a plant and mineral clay-based mask with a gentle electrical current, which feels like tiny needles on the skin, and helps to tone the hips and thighs and improve skin texture. Ideal for when you need a kick start into a new fitness regime, this is usually in the form of a course of six or 10 treatments.

water treatments

Water related spa treatments such as underwater hydrotherapy massage and blitz shower (high-pressure water jets that work on the lymphatic system) can help to eliminate fatty deposits and excess water to tone the body and boost circulation.

skin firming creams

While nothing replaces the all-round benefits of exercise, skin-firming body lotions can give a psychological lift to those bits of the body that need it most, helping to temporarily tighten and smooth the skin's surface. But don't expect miracles. It takes at least six weeks (or to the end of most bottles) before you'll notice a difference, if any, but skin will undoubtedly look and feel smoother to the touch; and the mere fact that you are regularly massaging something into the hip and thigh area has a positive uplifting effect.

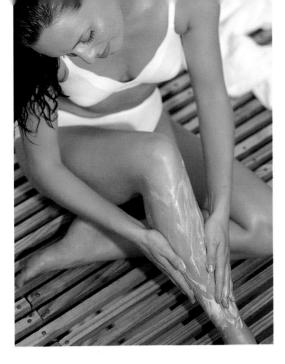

The bottom line

Ultimately the way to get a better body is through proper diet and exercise. US dermatologist Dr Karen Burke believes that you should be realistic about your body and set goals that are attainable. A better understanding of how your body works will encourage you to look at your lifestyle and take active steps to change harmful habits.

■ **Cellulite** is the term given to the dimpled, orange-peel look most women get on their thighs, bottom, and sometimes on the upper arms. It is said to affect around 80 per cent of women, of all shapes and sizes and levels of fitness but not, on the whole, men. The cause is not known, but the theory is that cellulite relates directly to the level of the female hormone oestrogen, which is why it often hits hardest during puberty and pregnancy. Many experts believe that cellulite is a sign of long-term imbalances within the body, and can be improved by cutting down on your consumption of fatty and sugary foods, drinking more water to flush out toxins, and boosting the circulation and the lymphatic system with regular exercise and manual massage.

■ **The lymphatic system** is our internal waste removal system. Lymph, the fluid that circulates around the body, picks up waste and toxins and deposits them in the lymph glands. A build up of waste due to poor circulation results in fatigue, water retention and poor circulation.

■ **Toxins** are poisons to the system: most notably alcohol, stress, smoke, pollution, pesticides and food additives. An overload results in poor skin and fatigue, which can eventually lead to bowel, bladder, liver and kidney problems.

■ **Detoxification** literally means removing these toxins from your body. A toxic overload results from a long list of these daily poisons and skin, hair and nails are the first areas to show the signs. Health experts recommend regular detoxing for a couple of days a month, by drinking plenty of mineral water, avoiding wheat and dairy foods, and practising deep breathing exercises to calm and relax the system.

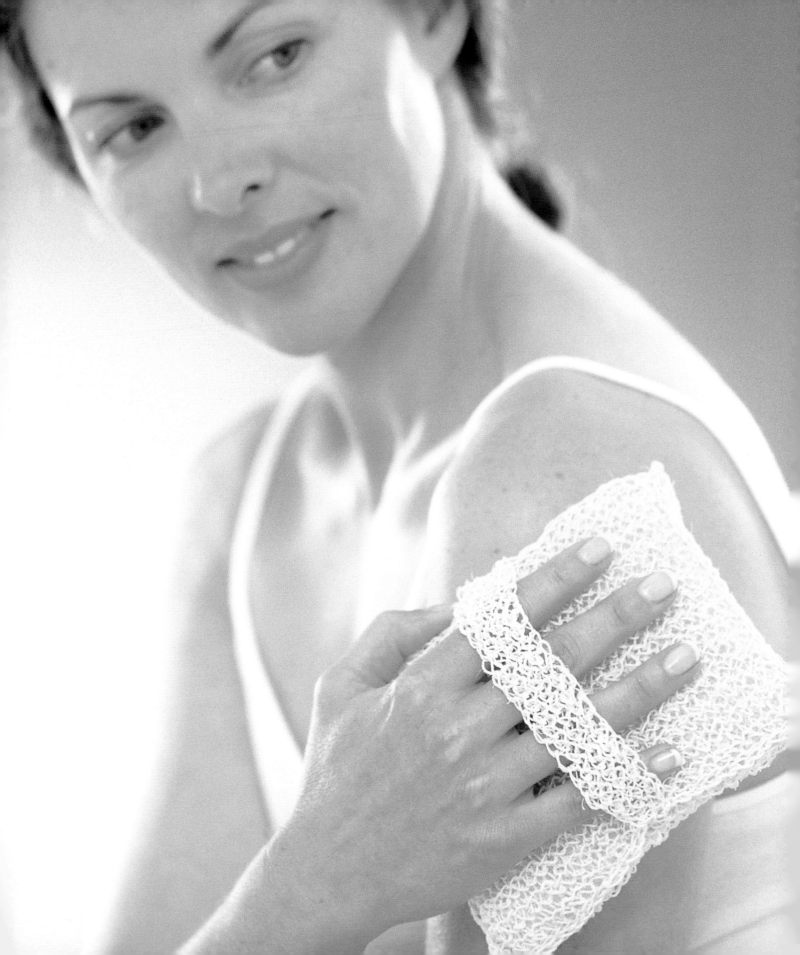

specialist
bodycare

Bodycare rituals today go way beyond basic hygiene. As spa treatments become more popular, reap the benefits of those you can try at home as a treat for you and your body.

body scrub

It's cathartic. Think of a body exfoliator as a really deep cleanse for your skin, helping to get rid of any dry or bumpy patches. Neglected skin, particularly on the backs of arms and the bottom, really responds well to a little extra attention and can be improved almost overnight. Choose from a basic loofah or mitt (brush over wet skin, rinse and pat dry with a towel); or scrub damp skin with a handful of coarse sea salt from the kitchen cupboard. Oil and salt scrubs are very popular and leave skin smooth and moisturised. While on the beach, sand is one of the best body exfoliators – and it's free.

who it's for

Everybody should scrub. It boosts circulation, improves skin tone and kicks the whole lymphatic system into action, which helps to eliminate toxins from the body.

how to use

Once a week buff your body religiously (including hands and feet) to give skin that fresh, glowing, 'polished' gleam that looks so healthy. Concentrate on the upper back, shoulders, bottom, elbows and knees, then treat everywhere else on the body with a light rub rather than a scrub. Amanda Birch, leading beauty therapist at Michaeljohn's Ragdale Clinic in London, recommends making your own oily salt rub. 'Get a handful of natural dead sea salts and mix together with plenty of pure almond or wheatgerm oil. With skin slightly damp, massage in the oil and salt together in a gentle circular movement all over the body. I like to add pine and juniper essential oils, for an uplifting smell that also helps to stimulate the circulation. Ideally stand over the bath so all the excess salt falls in the bath, then fill up a warm bath and soak in it afterwards to help detoxify the system.'

glorious mud

The healing properties of mud have been recognised for centuries and it is used in spa treatments for its deep cleansing, detoxifying benefits. These muds and clays are taken from the sea bed, including the Dead Sea, and from the earth. They contain minerals which are extremely therapeutic for skin health, especially in treating eczema and psoriasis. Salon mud body wraps involve being slathered in warm mud, wrapped up in layers of foil then wrapped in blankets to retain the heat and help draw out toxins. They are great whenever your body feels jaded, stressed or needs a good exfoliation, and are often used for slimming treatments, too, since they help the body eliminate toxins fast.

who they're for

All bodies can benefit from a mud wrap.

how to use

Be warned – a mud wrap can be messy. Try applying it while you're lying in a dry bath, or spread an old sheet on your bed, then make yourself comfortable and allow it to dry completely before rinsing it off. Your skin will look so much brighter. Try a mud bath at home. Mix Fuller's earth with warm water until it is muddy, but not runny, climb in and relax there for five minutes. Then every few days have another mud bath, increasing the length of time you spend in the bath to 15 minutes.

self tan

Many people believe that tanned skin makes us look slimmer and fitter than pale white skin, so be safe and fake it. Self-tanning products provide your skin with a tan without involving any of the sun's harmful effects. The lotions, creams and sprays are basically skin dyes, the majority of which contain the active ingredient dihy-droxyacetone (DHA), which reacts with skin's proteins (amino acids) in the outer layers of the skin to produce a browning effect. Many natural extracts are now being unearthed to stain the skin a natural colour, such as black walnut, mahakanni (an organic ingredient used in the East to colour the hair) and erythrulose (a natural sugar that adds a reddy brown tone to combat the yellowness of DHA). Most fake tans fade (usually over four days) as the skin flakes off, a process speeded up by scrubs, steam rooms and saunas.

Most lotions and sprays now are a great improvement on the traditional orange colour still associated with these products, and offer a 'nearly natural' tan in a matter of hours. But do practise applying them a few times, especially if you are very pale, and never try out a new formula the day before you go on holiday.

who they're for

Fake tan users fall into two different camps: those who want colour that's obvious – the 'if it doesn't show, why do it' philosophy. And there's the type who want the colour to be as subtle as possible, although still apparent, and preferably built up gradually. Allergic reactions to self-tans are rare, but if you have sensitive skin you should test a patch of skin first.

how to use

If you've yet to try using a self-tanning product, this is a foolproof method that suits even the whitest of skins. Start by exfoliating your body, then apply a moisturising cream to dry areas such as the elbows and knees, to act as a barrier. Now apply the self-tan all over, massaging it in evenly; leave it on for one hour, then have a shower. This ensures that any colour that hasn't been absorbed by this point will wash away, so you are less likely to end up with uneven patches. Many after-sun lotions now give

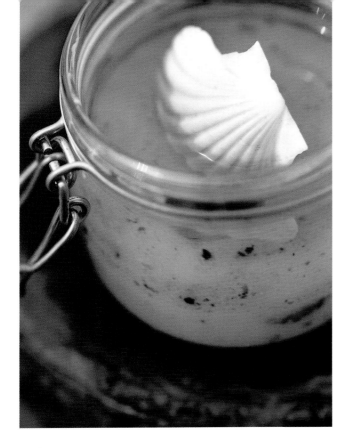

skin a subtle hint of colour too. These contain a tiny amount of DHA, so you can carry on using them as a daily body moisturiser, and they also give your skin a more subtle build up of colour over 48 hours.

seaweed

Seaweed (the generic name for marine algae) is known to have far- reaching benefits for our bodies. It contains a number of valuable minerals including iodine (which protects skin against premature ageing and keeps hair strong), sodium and potassium (which regulate cell fluid levels), iron (which improves the circulation), and copper (to maintain skin and muscle fibre). Because the oceans' waters and the plants which grow in them are so rich in minerals, seaweed and seawater-based body treatments and products have proven to be excellent at detoxifying the body, stimulating the metabolism and rejuvenating body and soul.

who they're for

Scientists have long known that the mineral content of seawater is almost identical to that of our bodies. In the 1900s, French biologist Rene Quinton discovered amaz-

ing similarities between our blood plasma and seawater, right down to their consistencies and mineral make-up (our white blood cells continue to live in seawater whereas they would die in any other medium). Hence the reason we have such an affinity with all things marine, and even those with chronic conditions such as arthritis can benefit.

how to use

From body washes, scrubs and lotions, to eye creams and body creams, marine extracts are now used in beauty products for their soothing, uplifting and healing properties, and to impart an overall feeling of well-being.

Use in the bath to unwind, detox and refresh. Lie with your body submerged for at least 10 minutes to allow the osmotic effect of the water to help draw out impurities. Freeze-dried seaweed, when mixed with water, turns into a warm. creamy mud mask which covers the body. Then as you lie wrapped in foil and covered in heated blankets, perspiration opens the pores and allows the seaweed's vitamins and minerals to be absorbed more effectively through the skin and into the bloodstream.

aromatherapy

Aromatherapy is the aromatic mind and body treatment that uses fragrant natural ingredients called pure essential oils – extracted from plants, flowers, fruits and the bark or resin of many trees – to heal ailments and restore emotional balance.

how it works

Essential oils give the aroma to a plant. They also contain dozens of complex chemicals with the power to affect the part of the brain which controls our memories and emotions, known as the lymbic system, through our sense of smell. These oils are easily absorbed through the skin and directly into the bloodstream. So whether you inhale them or rub them in, you can enhance your mood, beautify the skin and numb a headache in next to no time.

who it's for

Aromatherapy is beneficial to everyone for the mind, body and spirit. It can help with so many ailments from physical to psychological; particularly anxiety, insomnia, skin infections, hormonal imbalance and everyday muscular aches and pains. Even if you think you have never come across the oils before, you have experienced aromatherapy. Every time you peel an orange or slice a lemon, the zesty essential oil squirts out and evaporates into the air, waking you up and making you feel refreshed. Think then how therapeutic it would be to surround yourself with these oils in your daily life, affecting your mood at any given time, and relaxing or refreshing your senses whether at work or at home.

are essential oils safe?

Because of their potency, essential oils should be used in the correct concentration and never applied to the skin in their undiluted form: the only exceptions to this rule are lavender and tea tree oils. If you are pregnant or suffer from asthma, high blood pressure or epilepsy, always consult a qualified practitioner before using them. As with medicines, keep essential oils well out of the reach of children.

check the quality

The quality of essential oils varies hugely. Before buying, check that the label says 'pure essential oil'. If it also gives the plant derivative (the Latin name), the company probably takes the time to source the plant species, thereby providing good quality oil. And remember that pure essential oils are not oily! You can test the quality by putting a drop on a piece of paper – if there's an oily mark after a short while, the oil has been diluted with a vegetable oil, so it will not be as effective.

how to use them

The easiest and most beneficial ways to use the oils are in the bath, in a massage oil, or by inhaling them in a room vaporiser. But because they are so potent, most need to be diluted before you apply them to the skin.

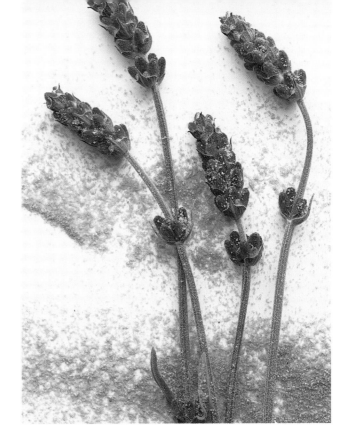

■ **Bath:** Use between six and 10 drops of pure essential oil, or one to two capfuls of a blend. Add to the bath once the water has run, then step in immediately.

■ **Massage:** Add five drops of your chosen oil to every 10ml (1tbsp) of carrier oil, such as sweet almond, wheat-germ or grapeseed oil. Rub between the hands, inhale, then massage into skin.

■ **Room vaporiser:** Add a few drops of oil to a bowl or warm water, or buy a vaporiser.

which oils to buy?

Choose an oil first and foremost for its smell. Aromatherapist Glenda Taylor says: 'It doesn't matter how therapeutic the oil might be, if you don't like the smell it won't have the same effect. The chances are that the oil whose smell you like the most is the one you really need there and then.' Here are six of the most useful oils:

■ **Lavender** is healing for minor cuts and burns.

■ **Geranium** acts as a sedative and a tonic, relieves anxiety and fatigue.

■ **Tea tree** is antiseptic, anti-viral and anti-bacterial, and heals cuts and grazes, insect bites and skin problems such as acne and athlete's foot.

■ **Peppermint** clears and refreshes the head and increases mental alertness.

■ **Rose** is sensual and emotionally uplifting, helps to boost confidence, beat stress and relieve tension. It's also great for dry, mature skins.

■ **Chamomile** calms the body and soothes minor skin irritations, including nappy rash.

Ancient aromas

The use of aromatic essences has been known to play a part in our lives from as far back as ancient Egyptian times. Records dating back to 4500BC reveal how perfumed oils, scented barks and resins were used in medicine, religion and in embalming.

But it wasn't until the beginning of this century that a French chemist called Dr Rene-Maurice Gattefossé actually created the name 'aromatherapy', following an incident where he burned his hand during a laboratory experiment and plunged it into the nearest vat of liquid, which just happened to contain lavender essential oil. Needless to say he was astounded at how quickly the pain was relieved and how his hand healed, and to this day lavender oil is considered to be the best first-aid kit to have to hand.

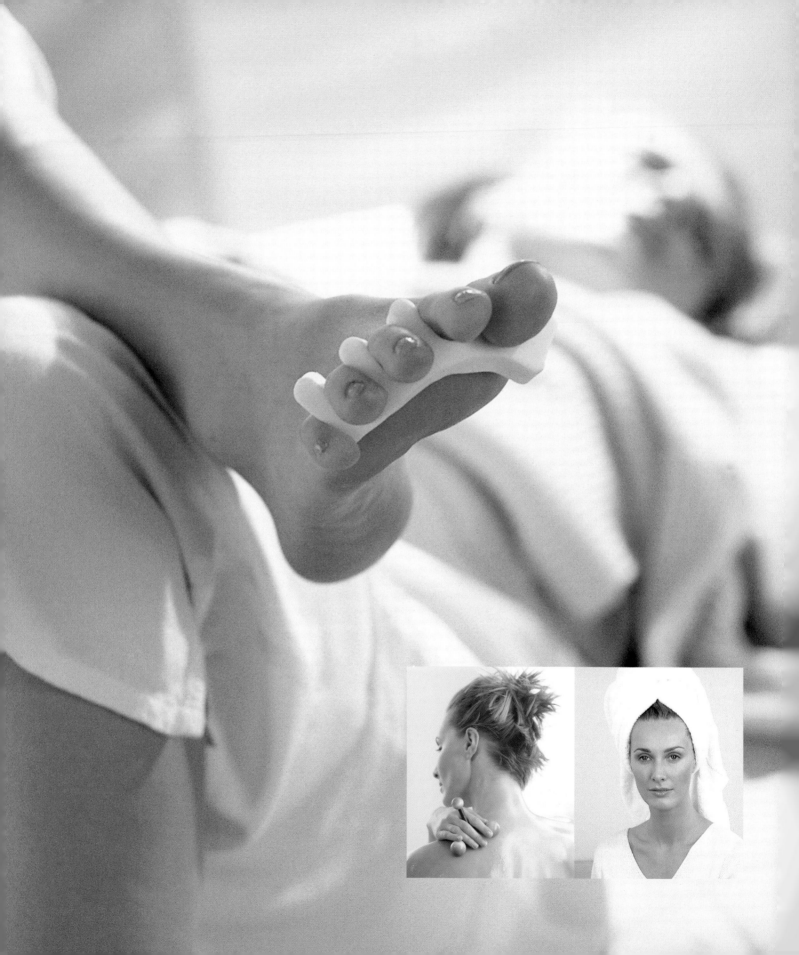

DIY home spa

It's easy to create a home spa experience. Use a room that's warm and has low lighting, and play relaxing music. Always make sure you have everything you need before you start.

Start with a salt body scrub Most professional body treatments now start with a gentle scrub. This not only helps to exfoliate dull skin, but also encourages any further treatment products to be better absorbed, making them more effective. Sea salt mixed with body oil is the most luxurious way to scrub, because it leaves skin so soft and smooth. Concentrate on your upper back and shoulders, buttocks, elbows, backs of upper arms and backs of legs.

Now have a long soak in the bath Don't underestimate the powerful effect of taking a bath; it's one of the best ways to detox your whole system as the osmotic effect of the bath water helps to draw out toxins. Beauty expert Liz Earle suggests adding 1kg of Epsom salts to the water to intensify the detoxifying effect. 'It will make you feel a floppy at first, but you'll soon feel energised.'

Try a little hydrotherapy After a long soak, create your own hydrotherapy treatment with the shower faucet. Change the water temperature to hot or cold, then spray vigorously with each setting for 10–20 seconds. Alternate six times. Finish with a warm spray for a few minutes. This gently mimics the ferocious Jet Douche treatment that you'd find in a health spa, which boosts circulation.

Create your own rose cocoon Inspired by an exclusive treatment at London's Spa NK, pamper yourself in layers of aromatic rose oil, rose mist and rose body cream. Spritz a little rosewater over your face and body, then add five drops of rose absolute to 10ml of sweet almond oil, and any basic barely-scented body cream that you have spare. Now massage in one layer after another, tuck yourself up in a warm blanket, and relax for 20 minutes.

Give yourself a scalp massage Sit up comfortably, close your eyes and relax the neck and shoulders. Gently rub tiny circles along your neck and up to the nape of your neck. Then press all along either side of your hairline, until you reach your centre parting. Now place all your fingers in your hair, gently massage the scalp, then lift the hair upwards in your fingers and pull ever so gently, for a count of three. Repeat several times. This is even nicer if someone else does it for you.

Treat your feet Practise walking around your home barefoot for at least 15 minutes, it's very therapeutic. Then give them a mini-facial. Start lavishing them with as many beauty products as you would your face. Use an exfoliatior around hard skin, soak in lavender oil, and add a moisturising face mask to keep feet smooth and soft.

your body

bust

Big or small, when it comes to breasts, we invariably want what we don't have. Advances in cosmetic surgery may make dreams come true for some, but it is better to look after what you've got.

good support

Breasts contain no muscular tissue and are literally suspended by the Coopers ligaments (which extend from the outer edges of the breasts to the nipples) and the pectoral muscles (which lie between the outer edges of the breasts and the armpits), so they need good support to help keep their shape and tone over the years. However, with age, gravity and breast-feeding, breasts often become pendulous as a result of over-stretched ligaments and over-stretched skin. After the menopause, when body fat is diminished, breasts lose their weight and elasticity, and sag.

how to care

Regularly massage in a little oil or cream to keep the skin on your breasts supple and elastic. Stretchmarks are common during puberty and pregnancy, and while you can't prevent them you may help to lessen the effect by keeping skin supple.

Breasts are fatty tissue and as such cannot be affected by exercise, although exercise to the pectoral muscles may improve the overall shape of the bust. However the skin around the throat supports the bust, so remember to carry your facial skincare over into this area. If your breasts feel very heavy, wear a lightweight bra at night.

instant remedies

■ **Invest in a good supportive bra.** It is always a good idea to be correctly fitted for a new bra. A good fit ensures that your breasts fill the cups without spilling over the top or at the sides, and the band underneath (whether wired or not) should support without digging in and sit comfortably across the centre of your back without riding up. If you find there are marks left on your breasts by your bra when you take it off at night, you need a bigger size.

■ **Start adopting a better posture now:** rounded shoulders equal a saggy bust.

■ **Apply a moisturiser or body oil** to the bust area daily. Keeping the skin here soft and supple will help it to maintain its elasticity.

■ **Try this exercise, while sitting or standing,** to tone the pectoral muscles. Clasp your hands and raise your elbows out in front you at shoulder level, six inches apart from each other. Squeeze elbows and forearms together as hard as you can, hold for a count of four. Repeat five times. Then bring your elbows together and raise your arms as high as you can over your head. Hold for a count of three. Repeat the whole sequence five times.

tummy

While the artist Rubens may have celebrated a rounded female belly, most women today would prefer to have a flat tummy. One joy of pregnancy is that for nine months you don't have to hold your tummy in – but then!

improve your posture

Few of us feel confident about our tummy; it's the one area of a woman's body that rarely seems ideal. And years of poor posture only serve to enhance a rounded tummy, since only a strong back will encourage a firmer stomach. Pull it in and stand tall – it'll make a huge difference to your overall shape as well as that of your tummy.

In pregnancy the skin and muscles around the tummy stretch way beyond belief, but with hard work it is possible to regain your shape; and children should never be the excuse for developing slack muscles and losing tone. It is important to persevere, because by keeping your stomach muscles fit and firm, you will help to prevent debilitating back pain later in life.

how to care

Exercise is the only way to improve your tummy. The best exercise for a flatter tummy is Pilates, which helps to stretch and strengthen specific muscle groups. With all abdominal exercises it is important to breathe correctly. Always take a deep breath in, then breathe out as you do the movement, holding your tummy in as you move. And remember, with all sit-up tummy exercises you shouldn't have to sit up from lying down or you will strain yourself. Research now shows that the smaller, slower and more accurate the movement, the more effective the exercise.

tummy tips

■ **Don't slouch** Whether you are walking, standing or sitting, you should try to keep your back in a straight line. Try this Pilates stretching technique, which helps to adopt a straighter back. Stand against a wall with your entire back pressed against it. Breathe in, and pull your tummy right in against the wall as you breathe out. Then slowly roll your neck and upper back downwards, as if you're lifting each vertebra off the wall as you roll down. Only go as far as is comfortable.

■ **Try to avoid carrying a toddler** otherwise we tend to curve the back and stick the tummy out to support the extra weight, developing bad posture, when we should be pulling it all in.

■ **Sleep on a soft mattress** on a firm base, not a sprung mattress. This is the best type of bed for anyone with back problems.

■ **Instant remedies** Sorry, but there just aren't any! Firming your tummy takes time, but it's definitely worth it.

■ **Tighten up** Look for 'knicker grippers', the best high-waisted tummy control underwear with Lycra, to hold everything firmly in place.

legs

We run, walk and stand with them, yet we rarely feel as confident as we should about our legs. Swollen ankles, fluid retention and varicose veins may become more common with age, but there's plenty we can do to help.

why legs develop problems

Lack of circulation is the biggest threat to having lovely legs and keeping them that way. A sedentary lifestyle spent sitting at a desk for long periods of time or driving the children back and forth to school, means that circulation is constantly restricted, which can cause problems with veins. And as you get older, swollen ankles become increasingly common, along with varicose veins which are most commonly caused by weight gain.

how to care

Pay particular attention to the way you treat your legs. Regular exercise boosts circulation and will help prevent varicose veins from occurring. Avoid standing for long periods of time or sitting with your legs crossed. Put your feet up at regular intervals, especially if you are pregnant. Look at taking supplements that stimulate circulation, such as ginkgo biloba and silica.

Try giving your legs a daily stimulating massage, using firm strokes while massaging in your body lotion. Start with the soles of your feet, applying gentle pressure to the arch of your foot and between your toes. Now gently stroke your legs upwards from the ankle to the knee, finishing with firm pressure behind the knee.

leg revivers

■ **If you suffer from small spider veins** on your legs, especially around the ankles, knees and inner thighs, a simple treatment called sclerotherapy, which involves injecting a solution in the vein to seal the vein off, helps to diminish their appearance. However, while many beauty salons may offer this procedure, it should only be carried out by a qualified doctor.

■ **For tired, aching legs,** Aromazone is a fantastic half-hour salon treatment. It uses inflatable boots that cover each leg and compress them from the ankle to thigh in a rhythmical action. The effect is extremely uplifting.

■ **Massage your legs** Mix 10 ml jojoba oil with four drops each of peppermint and lavender essential oils, then massage in daily to wake up weary legs.

■ **For pale legs** Use fake tan to make them look and feel fitter and more bare-able.

■ **In the heat,** use a spritzer or foot spray to cool legs down fast.

■ **Exercise your legs** Either sitting or standing: with your feet flat on the floor, lift your toes up towards you, keeping your heels flat on the floor. Lower your toes and with a rolling action, lift your heels up. Repeat 15–20 times.

feet

Don't ignore them. They carry us around with them all day long, invariably bound up in ill-fitting shoes, get virtually ignored and then we wonder why they start to complain! Time to give them some attention.

why feet are sensitive

Richly supplied with over 70,000 nerve endings in each foot, our feet are one of the most sensitive and responsive parts of the body. As evidence, rub an onion on the soles of your feet and within moments you will taste it on your breath. The diagnostic therapy reflexology uses massage and finger pressure on the soles of the feet to help stimulate specific energy points and restore energy flow throughout the body.

how to care

Get into the habit of a little bit of daily TLC immediately following a bath or shower, and you'll soon notice results. Start off by lavishing your feet with as many leftover, never-got-around-to-finishing-them, face and body beauty products that you can muster up. Exfoliators, face masks, creams and potions work just as well on your feet as they do on your face.

Try giving yourself a foot massage for just five minutes while you wait for your body lotion to sink in. Rub a couple of drops of body oil between the palms of your hands, smooth over your foot then make long, firm thumb sweeps along the length of the sole of the foot from the arch to the toes. Next, make small circles using your thumbs, working from the ball of the foot to the heel. Finally, hold the toes with one hand and the heel with the other and wring the foot by twisting your hands in opposite directions.

pamper your feet

■ **Always paint your toenails,** especially if you don't like your feet, because it focuses on them and always manages to make them look prettier.

■ **The most relaxing treat** – simply because it makes you sit back and unwind for 10 minutes – is to soak your feet in a bowl of warm water with a couple of drops of geranium and lavender essential oils to soothe and relax aching arches after a long day.

■ **A paraffin hand and foot treatment,** favoured at health spas, is one of the best ways to soften and smooth dry skin on hands and feet. Warm wax is painted on to the skin, then hands and feet are wrapped up to keep them warm and to help absorb moisture. When they're removed your skin is dewy soft and glistening, and your cuticles look clean and smooth.

■ **If your feet are really dry,** the best treatment is to smother them in Vaseline, wrap them up in old socks and leave these on all night. An old Chinese remedy, it's not recommended on hot summer nights, but it's guaranteed to improve the roughest of feet by morning.

body solutions

Tried and tested remedies for some common problems.

■ **If you have sunburn,** have a cool bath and add three drops of chamomile oil and five drops of lavender oil to soothe and heal delicate skin.

■ **If your toenails are less than perfect,** try giving them a French manicure finish (white painted nail tips and pale pink polish over the top) to help even out nail lengths and give the illusion of prettier toes.

■ **If you find it hard to sleep,** try this soporific aromatherapy blend massage on the neck and chest and breathe in the vapour. Add two drops of frankincense oil and one drop each of lavender, marjoram and sandalwood oils to 10ml of sweet almond oil.

■ **If you suffer from puffy ankles,** give them a soak. Immerse your feet up to the ankles in hot and then cold water to help reduce swelling fast. Then put your feet up to improve circulation.

■ **If you often feel tired or lethargic** you may lack essential B vitamins, magnesium and iron. Try eating several low-fat snacks throughout the day, and avoid quick boosters such as caffeine or sweets, which only exacerbate fatigue over time

■ **If your skin is dry,** add 10ml of sweet almond oil to your bath water along with your favourite essential oil

■ **If you suffer from goose flesh,** you need a daily circulation booster to kick start your system back into action. Dry body brushing (see p.64) is very effective, or use a body exfoliator in the bath or shower, such as a loofah or body scrub.

■ **If your neck feels tense,** slowly turn your head to the left as far as you can stretch and hold for a count of 10. Then turn back to face the centre and slowly drop your head down to your chest; hold for 10 then bring your head up again. Now turn your head to the right as far as you can stretch and hold for 10. Repeat 5 times in a row.

■ **If your muscles ache after a workout,** soak in a warm bath filled with two drops of black pepper essential oil, three drops of frankincense oil and one drop of rose oil.

■ **If you suffer from bad breath,** take vitamin C and calcium supplements, chew on a bit of parsley, bump up your intake of live yoghurt and drink peppermint tea.

■ **When you need a pick-me-up,** try one of these energising essential oil baths. Add either two drops each of basil, clary sage and thyme oil, or two drops of peppermint and four drops of rosemary.

■ **If you suffer from cellulite and poor circulation,** try experimenting with herbal teas. Not only will you cut down on your caffeine intake, many teas such as dandelion (for the liver) and nettle (for the blood) are a good natural tonic for a sluggish system.

■ **Be good to yourself.** Author Louise Hay, in her book *You Can Heal Your Life,* believes that many physical problems relate to our emotional state. Feeling deprived and denying yourself small treats in life (such as that morning cappuccino) won't make you feel good about yourself. 'All things in moderation' and 'a little of what you fancy' are the key to better living.

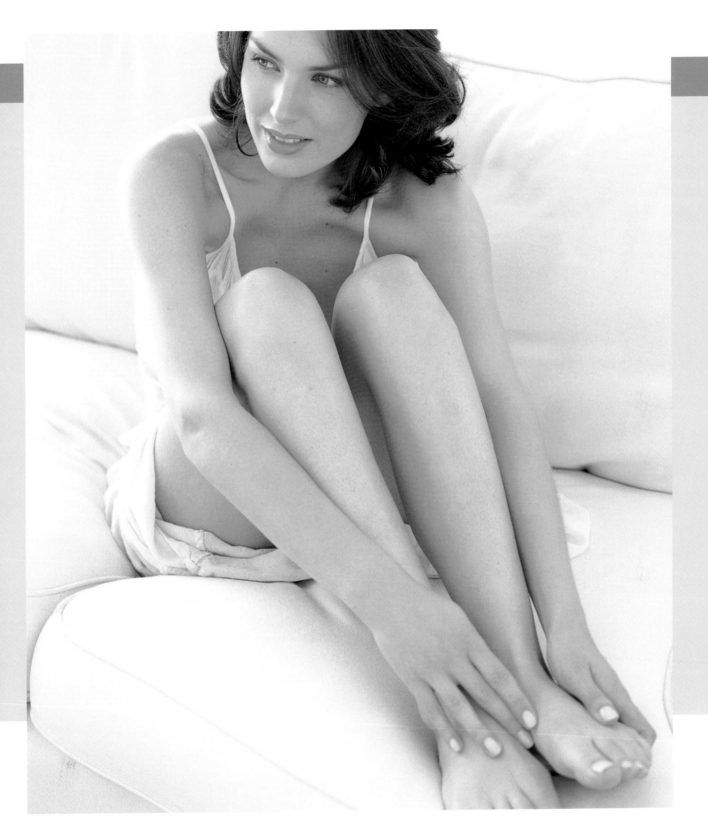

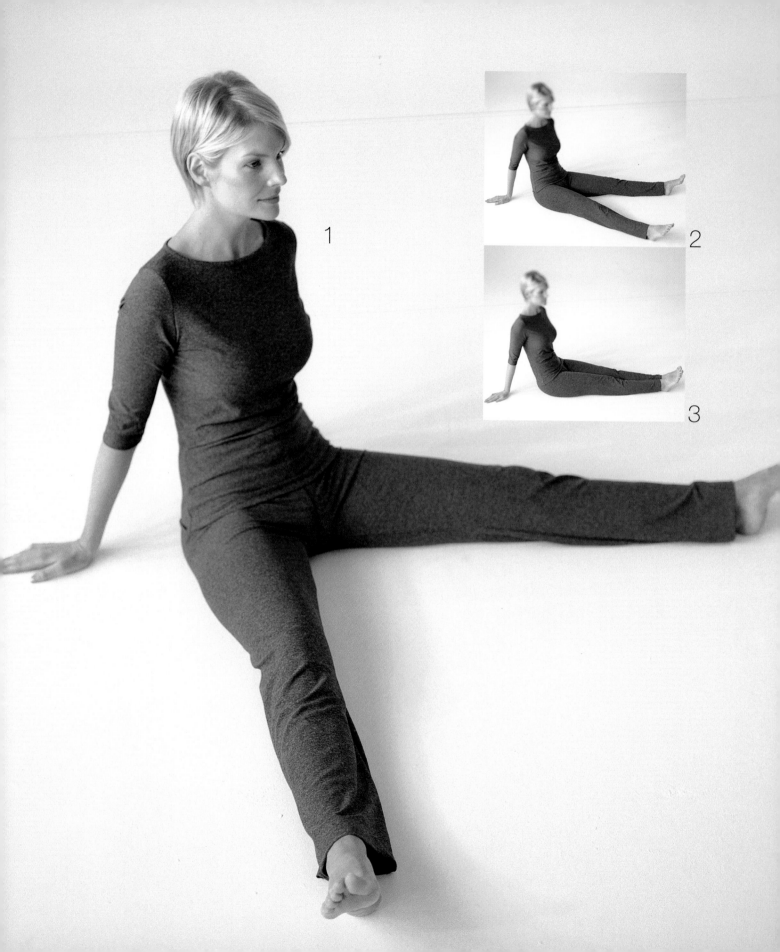

1

2

3

anti-ageing body workout

To increase your suppleness and body tone and improve your posture, try this short introduction to Pilates devised by leading expert Alan Herdman.

inner thighs

Get into position Sit on the floor with legs stretched out comfortably to the sides and feet flexed with relaxed toes. Place your hands on the floor behind you, keeping elbows soft to avoid tension, then lean back slightly (as if leaning into a sofa behind you). This allows you to use your tummy muscles rather than your hips and also means your tummy is supporting you and not your back. Keep shoulders slightly back from your hips and square with the floor [1].

Now move Breathe in and 'pull navel to spine' (see box below for explanation), hold your tummy in as you gently breathe out and slowly slide your right leg across to meet with your left leg [2]. Concentrate on using the inner thigh muscle to bring your leg across and not your knee or whole leg. Breathe in with legs together [3], pull navel to spine, then breathe out and return to original position. Alternate legs and repeat 10 times each side.

Pilates

Pilates is a body-conditioning technique created over 40 years ago by Joseph Pilates, a German athlete. With elements of t'ai chi, yoga and the Alexander technique, Pilates works by combining strict posture and breathing techniques to produce greater body awareness, self-discipline and inner relaxation. It works by stretching (and thereby elongating) the muscles, rather than building them up, working against resistance and without gravity, so each exercise is safe for all ages and all levels of fitness.

■ Correct breathing works the lungs and heart, boosts blood circulation and makes it much easier to control tension. Always breathe in before each movement, and out during it.

■ 'Pull navel to spine' is a phrase used with every Pilates exercise and ensures that you are making the most of each movement. It simply means pull your tummy in from your belly button, as far in as you can, as if it will touch your spine. You should keep holding your tummy in like this throughout the whole movement.

■ Wear loose comfortable clothing and keep feet bare or in socks.

waist side bends

1 **2**

side abdominals

1

2

3

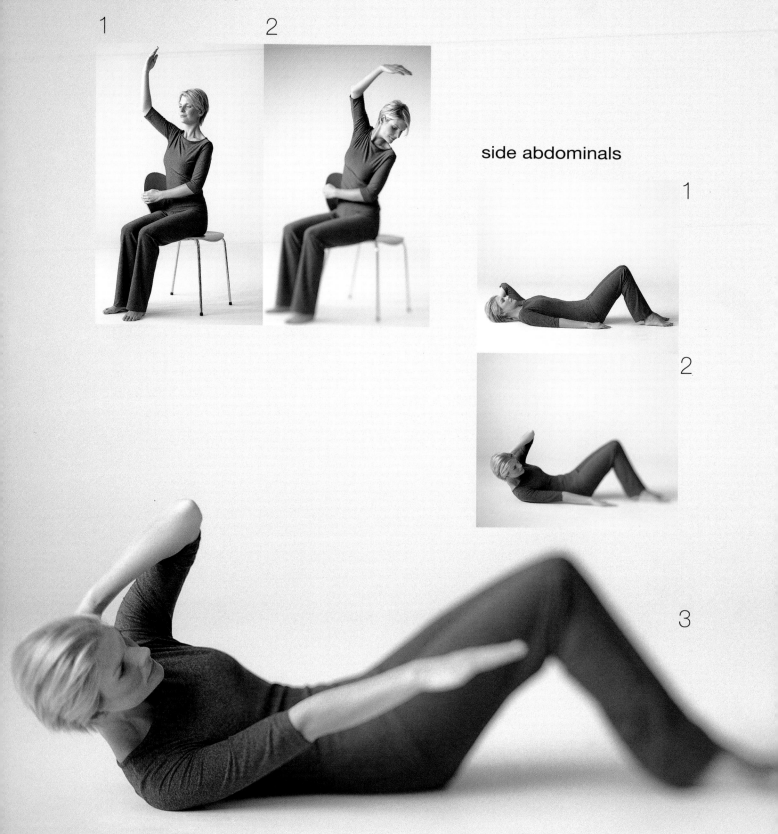

side abdominals

Get into position Lie down flat with knees bent and feet flat, then place your left hand under your head and right arm along the floor with palm facing down [1].

Now move Breathe in, pull navel to spine, then breathe out as you slowly come up, lifting your left side up and across [2]. Imagine that someone is lifting you up from under your shoulder blade to increase the lift, using the tummy muscles to do the work rather than the arm. If you feel tension in the neck, give it more support with both hands, then raise your right arm up alongside your knee [3]. Repeat 10 times each side.

waist side bends

Get into position Sit upright and sideways on a dining chair with knees hip width apart. Pull up through the centre of your upper body as if there's a string pulling your head up. Gently bend your right arm and place above your head with the left arm bent slightly in front [1]. Keep arms soft and relaxed with no tension in the neck.

Now move Breathe in, pull navel to spine, and breathe out as you bend over to one side. Go as far as you can comfortably reach, feeling the stretch, and hold for a count of four [2]. Breathe in, pull navel to spine and breathe out to come back upright. Repeat 10 times each side.

buttock squeeze

(not shown)

Get into position Lie face down on the floor with your head resting on your forearms. Place a pillow under the tummy to support the lumbar spine (the curve) and a small rolled towel under both knees. Think of your tailbone (sitting bone) being pulled towards your feet, and keep your feet relaxed throughout.

Now move Breathe in, pull navel to spine, and breathe out as you squeeze the buttocks together and slowly lift the left leg. Bring your lower leg upright, keeping the foot relaxed, otherwise you use the calf muscles rather than the thigh and hamstring. Hold for a count of four, then release. Repeat 10 times.

your make-up

with the power to smooth,

soften and prettify your

looks, make-up is an

indispensable beauty tool

for all ages. Once you've

mastered the art of your

own make-up essentials, real

beauty becomes timeless

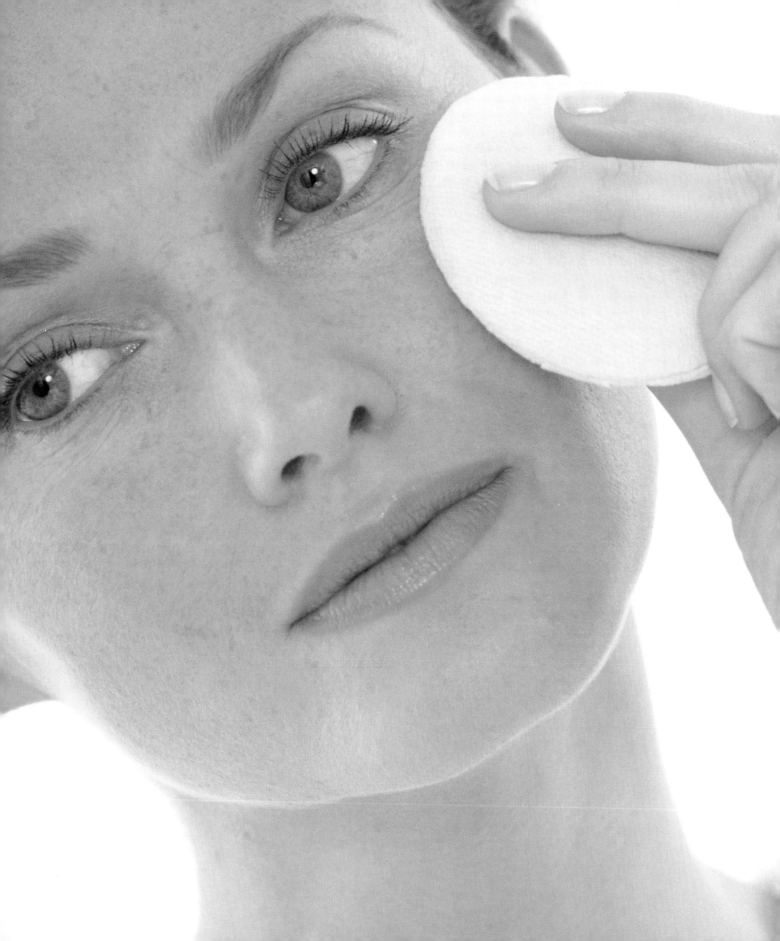

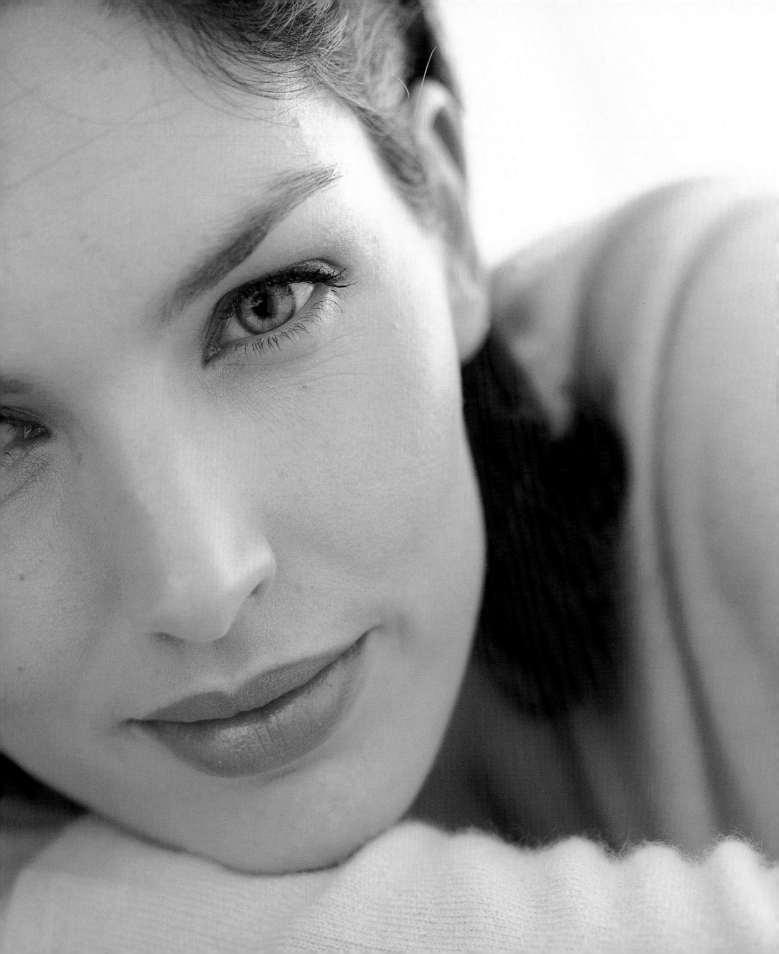

how make-up rejuvenates

make-up for all ages

Make-up is to be enjoyed at any age, and the way you wear it says much about how you feel. By your 40s you are confident enough to wear it to feel fabulous, not impress others.

As everything in your life changes from month to month, season to season, so too should your make-up. Life doesn't stand still, so why should you? As a rule, make-up isn't known for its rejuvenating effect on the skin. Applied badly it can sink into creases, accentuate fine lines and make you wish you hadn't bothered in the first place. When you reach this point in your make-up history, you need to follow the golden rule: less is more.

in your 20s

You can wear any make-up; any vibrant colour and shiny texture. You can even overdo it and still get away with it because your skin looks fresh and young and at this point in your life make-up is for fun.

in your 30s

Things are becoming a little less radiant at this point in life. Your skin is still firm and relatively smooth, but all those parties and late nights have started to take their toll, and you're needing more radiance-boosting colour and camouflage concealer to add to your make-up repertoire. Bold colour now begins to feel a little too showy and although you like your make-up to look modern and fresh, you are happiest mixing new textures and colours with a good base in which you feel confident.

in your 40s

You know your face and what suits you, and are more confident about who you are. You no longer need to wear make-up to be 'in', but more to perfect your features, which are just starting to lose their youthful bloom. Your skin is showing its first few lines around the eyes and forehead, and blusher becomes your number one ally as it puts back the colour in your cheeks that has started to fade.

in your 50s and beyond

Less is most definitely more. As brows and lashes fade along with your hair colour, so too does your skin tone pale. Subtlety is the key. Where once you wore black mascara, now you should wear a natural-looking brown. And where you wore pink blusher, now make it a softer tawny pink. Your skin has more wrinkles and the overall skin texture has slackened. Now's the time to be careful about the make-up base you use. Avoid a matte texture, which flattens and deadens mature skins, and steer clear of very shiny textures too, which highlight any skin that isn't smooth. Stick to semi-sheer, semi-matte textures for foundation, powders and lipsticks which make skin look like skin, only more radiant.

the magic of make-up

The pure pleasure and playfulness of applying make-up should make you feel as good as you look. Think back to a little girl's first brush with powder and lipstick at her mother's dressing table: it was a magical moment. But somehow, somewhere along the line, we begin to lose the delight. Once make-up becomes a practical, everyday, repetitive occurrence, the joy is gone. Yet there has never been a more creative era in cosmetics. Today, you can buy every conceivable colour and texture, no matter what your skin tone, from iridescent silk powders to the sheerest shadows and seductive glosses imaginable. So start to imagine …

stuck in a rut?

It's acknowledged that the one way a woman can truly age herself is with her make-up. Being comfortable with a look is one thing, but sticking with it for an entire decade is quite another. However, old make-up habits are hard to break. That basic brown contouring eyeshadow may have served you well, but in the three years

you've had it (any longer and for pure hygiene's sake you'd better throw it away now), your skin tone may have changed, your face shape may have become leaner with age – and the chances are you haven't taken the time to stop, look in a mirror and take note of how your make-up looks today as opposed to way back then.

have a makeover

As you get older your face shape, skin texture and colouring change, so you will undoubtedly need to revise your make-up on a regular basis. Indeed it is often when we fail to register subtle changes in the way we look that we first start to become stuck in a make-up rut. The best way to rejuvenate your looks is with a professional make-up lesson from an experienced make-up artist.

Either visit the counter of a particular brand that you like and can identify with (do the beauty consultants reflect the way you'd like to look?) or contact a make-up artist through an agency. There are pros and cons for both. A make-up lesson at the counter is invariably free and lasts around 15 minutes, but you may well feel compelled to buy something on the spot and they will only promote the one brand. A professional make-up artist booked through an agency may prove to be quite expensive (often in excess of £200 for a couple of hours), but the advice is totally unbiased and you will learn a great deal from the experience.

make-up essentials

There are a few select items of make-up that are so indispensable that virtually every woman can use them. Just take your pick:

■ **Concealer** Yellow-toned to blend in best with your skintone. Top of the list: Laura Mercier Secret Concealer.

■ **Foundation** to smooth, even and perfect every skin. In every conceivable colour: Prescriptives Virtual Skin.

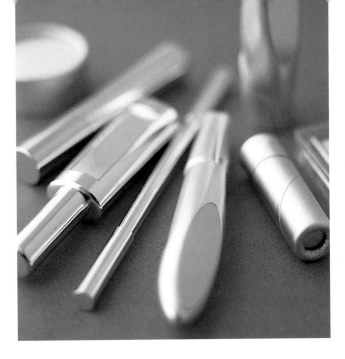

Loose Powder Superfine for the sheerest, most ageless, barely-there finish imaginable. Finest by far: Shiseido's The Make-up Silk Powder

Blusher The perfect neutral pinky beige that imitates a bracing walk in the fresh air. Suits most skins: Helena Rubinstein Colour Fusion Blush in Rosebud.

Black mascara A glossy, sheer formula that enhances the eyelashes without making them look too intense. Make-up artists' all-time favourite: Maybelline Great Lash Mascara.

Brow pencil that is waxy so it doesn't smudge, but still blends well. Hot favourite: Laura Mercier Brow Pencil.

Mid brown eye-shadow that's a neutral shade to help shape and contour the eyes. Famously fabulous: MAC Taupe Eyeshadow.

White eye-shadow to highlight and illuminate the eyes, and to help shape and enhance darker areas. Picked by the pros: MAC White Eyeshadow.

Lipliner Use to shade your lips rather than line them, otherwise it will only leave an old-fashioned rim to your lips. Best neutral colour: MAC Spice Lip Pencil.

Clear lip gloss that also serves as the best lip balm, and can be mixed with your favourite creamy lip colour to create a more glossy, sheer texture. Cheapest by far: Vaseline Petroleum Jelly.

Stay looking modern

Less is more. If you were to apply make-up to every feature at the same time, you'd soon look overdone. Make-up artist Stephane Marais recommends choosing a look that focuses on one great feature.

If you like your mouth, enhance your lips with a darker colour, and go lighter on your eyes.

If you like your eyes, enhance them with liner and shadow, and go lighter on your lips.

If you like your cheekbones, emphasise your cheeks and brows for a very natural, groomed look, and play down your lips and eyes.

Stick to neutral, natural shades of make-up that complement your skin tone rather than vivid colours that invariably look too harsh on skins over 30.

Go for texture that flatters the skin. Keep it matte along the T-zone and shimmery on the cheeks, temples and browbones (where there are also fewer creases and wrinkles). Always keep an eye on what's in fashion, then play it down by adding just one element to your usual make-up, such as pink gloss or smoky eyes.

make-up tricks

■ **'To make the whites of your eyes appear brighter,** use a light blue pencil under the eyes.' says make-up artist Roxanne New. 'Soft blue eye-shadow lightly dusted under the eyes works well too.'

■ **'Scrub yellow, discoloured nails** with the juice of a fresh lemon. Then swipe a white pencil under your nail tips to boost their brightness.' Top London manicurist and nail technician Iris Chapple.

■ **If lipstick is on your teeth,** do what models do. After applying your lipstick, place your index finger in your mouth, close your lips around it and pull your finger out. Any lipstick that would have ended up on your teeth instantly comes off on your finger.

■ **'If you're in a rush,** apply a neutral pinky brown lip colour rather than red or other deep-coloured lipsticks, which require more lengthy and precise application.' `Make-up artist Maggie Hunt.

■ **'Wear an apricot blusher** to make skin look more radiant.' Olivier Echaudemaison of Guerlain.

■ **'For a modern, quick make-up** that doesn't break the bank, just use mascara and lip gloss. The mascara will lengthen the lashes and accentuate the eyes. The lip gloss can be used sparingly on eyelids and cheeks as well as on the lips, if applied with your fingertips, and adds a youthful sheen to skin.' Fred Farrugia of Lancôme.

■ **When applying powder around the mouth area,** blow out your cheeks so that less powder collects in the creases.

■ **'Using shadow along the lash line** creates a softer eyeline on older skin than pencil or liquid, and is much easier to control.' Make-up artist Bobbi Brown.

■ **Prepare your skin for make-up.** Spritz clean complexion with a facial mist before applying moisturiser. This will give skin a boost and help to soften fine lines prior to applying make-up.

■ **Lips often thin with age.** For the quickest lip plump, simply apply a little gloss on the centre of the bottom lip. Pale lip colours make lips seem bigger; avoid dark colours which make them appear thinner still.

■ **'If your concealer makes your eyes appear more tired,** crepey or baggy, its texture is probably too heavy and is dragging your skin down. And if your skin is also dry, you may need to apply eye cream underneath. Apply only a little and make sure that it is well absorbed (preferably with a matte finish) so concealer looks smooth when applied on top.' Bobbi Brown.

■ **'To check how perfectly you have drawn your lips,** wrap a cotton pad in a tissue and blot your lips with the pad. Match up the outline to see just how exact they are.' Estée Lauder.

■ **'Instead of using an eyeliner sharpener,** sharpen eye pencils with a razor blade, shaving repeatedly from top to bottom on one side and then again on the opposite side. The result is a rectangular tip that allows for a cleaner line between the lashes.' American make-up artist Laura Mercier.

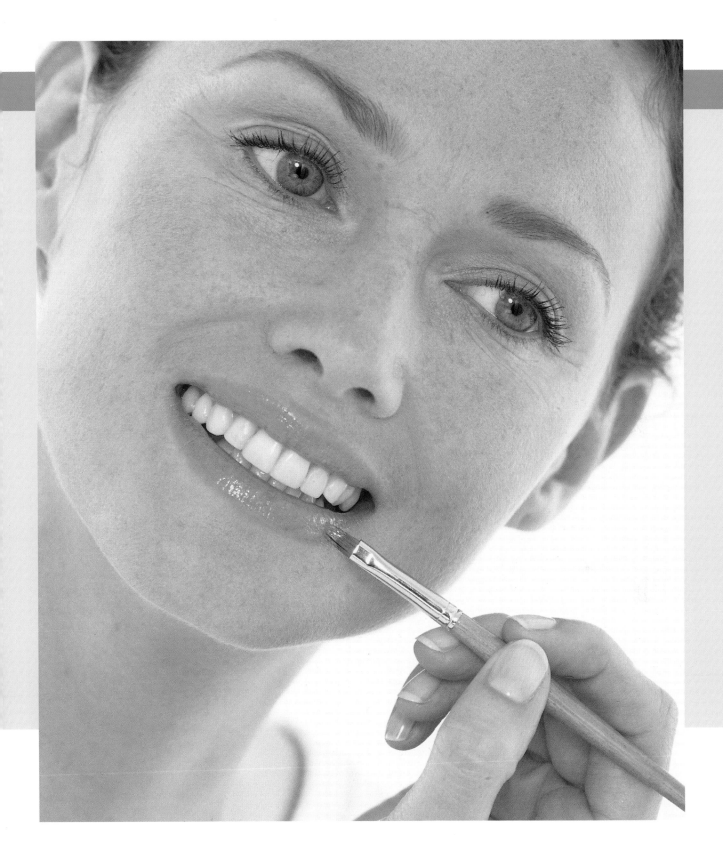

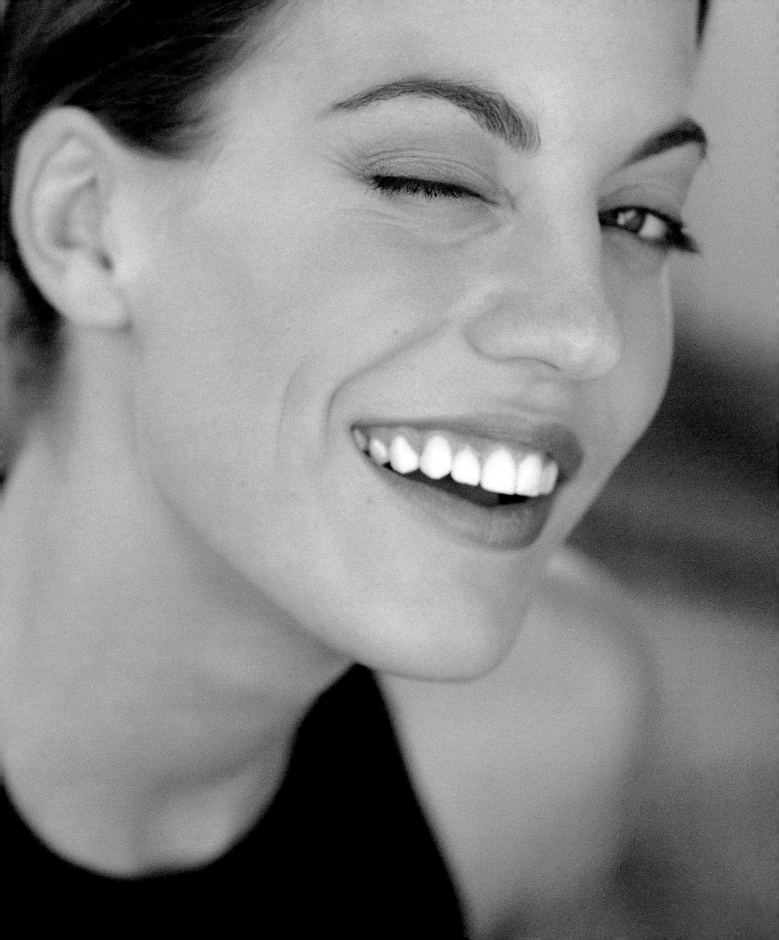

daily make-up requirements

why make-up matters

The best of allies, make-up has the power to boost your confidence, send your spirits soaring, and make you feel sexy and self-assured, with just one sweeping gesture.

what make-up does

The 'right' make-up is different for every woman. To one, it may be a full make-up worn daily to project a professional, groomed image. To another, it may be just a slick of lip gloss and a dusting of blusher before dashing to drop the children off at school – if she has the time, of course. But ultimately, the answer is that your make-up should be whatever you need it to be. It should enhance and perfect all that Mother Nature gave you.

The best make-up will never dramatically change your looks, only help you look better – more radiant and more youthful. Make-up trends change so fast these days that you barely have time to catch on to a new thing before it's been and gone. In the past we could stick with a look for a decade (think 50s eyeliner, followed by the 60s passion for creamy frosted eye-shadow) and still get away with being stylish and modern.

stick to what suits you

Now, no sooner has lilac become trendy, but blue is back, and gold is waiting on the horizon for its magical 'modern' moment in fashion. What we all seem to forget while trying to keep up, is what actually suits us – our colouring and our lifestyle. Sure, sometimes something amazing comes along and it becomes a firm favourite in your make-up bag for what seems like forever, but ultimately you should never lose sight of you. The art of perfecting you and you alone: that is what make-up is for. If you must be a slave to fashion, then change the colour of your nail polish daily, revamp your lip colour, but otherwise leave everything else to the teenagers: you just don't need it any more.

The right cosmetics applied correctly add the finishing touch to your looks. It doesn't have to take much to bring out the best in your face, but learning how to use cosmetics effectively takes a little practise and a bit of know-how.

foundation

Very few of us have perfect flawless skin, but that doesn't mean we can't come closer to it. Clear, smooth skin is considered the beauty ideal, and the best way to achieve it is by applying a good foundation.

how to wear it

The way we wear foundation has evolved over the years, from the all-over artificial, mask-like make-up our mothers wore, to an invisible, barely-there, sheer layer applied only in those areas where you need it, rather than all over as before. 'The most common mistake women make is to use too much foundation and the wrong shade,' says Laura Mercier.

what texture?

There are many different foundation textures to choose from; the best one to use depends on your particular skin type and what finish you are looking for. Two-in-one powder foundations (also called cream-to-powder) are speedy compact formulas which give a matte, dry, powdery finish. Great if you're on the run, these are ideal for normal to oily skins but dry, mature skins may find them too drying.

Stick foundations are convenient and easy to use – just dot where you need cover, a bit like concealer. Again, dry skins suit these the least, but provided you prime your skin well beforehand with moisturiser and blend well, they give great coverage and are very popular. Satin foundations (also called semi-matte or demi-matte) are often liquid foundations that give a natural, light cover and suit pretty much all skin types. Some may contain light-diffusing pigments: these reflect the light, giving the illusion of flawless, younger looking skin and are ideal for more mature skin types. Oil-free foundations are designed for those with oily skin. They are usually water-based and contain tiny silicone particles to help them stay on the skin.

how to apply

First, prime the skin with moisturiser and allow it to become fully absorbed (up to 15 minutes), then blot off any excess before applying foundation. Laura Mercier is the queen of the flawless base. She recommends only applying foundation where you need to even out skin tone, not necessarily over the entire face. This will keep your make-up looking more fresh, modern and youthful. If you are going to use a sponge, Laura recommends using it damp. 'Make sure any excess water has been squeezed out and work the foundation into the sponge well, so that the application is light and even and not streaky. If you can't see it going on your skin you've got the right shade and you're doing it right.'

Never put too much foundation around the eyes, otherwise it will emphasise fine lines and wrinkles. Don't layer too many different bases, either, says Laura. If you know you will be using a concealer, don't use foundation around the eye area, but remember to apply foundation to the ears, which are often slightly redder than the face. Always apply base by a window, so that you are in natural light. And the magical secret, as every make-up artist will tell you, is blend, blend, blend.

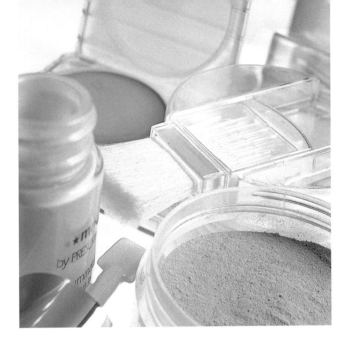

which colour?

This is the hardest part to get right. Most women are not clear what colour their skin really is, often believing it to be pinkish when it is actually more yellow. Bobbi Brown was one of the first experts to come up with her own range of yellow-based foundations, which are much more flattering than more traditional pinky shades.

Make this your number one rule: foundation should never add colour to your skin. It should blend in with your natural skin tone along the jawline, next to the neck. To find the right colour for you, test a shade there. If it vanishes onto your skin, you've found the perfect colour match. Never go darker with colour: it will be impossible to blend and you will be left with a tell-tale tide mark. Always choose a new foundation in natural daylight. Department stores are renowned for having poor lighting, and you can be sure that what may look like the right colour at the cosmetics counter is nowhere near the one you really need. Once you've tested a colour on your face, go and look at it in the daylight. Never feel rushed or pressurised into buying foundation. It is the single most transforming item of make-up, and is worth getting right.

which brush?

Make-up artists always apply foundation with a cosmetic sponge wedge because it is more hygienic for them to use on models' faces than their own fingertips. However most would agree that, provided they're clean, your fingers provide the very best way to apply foundation, enabling you to reach the tiniest of corners that a sponge can't reach and letting you work it into your skin, thereby avoiding streaking.

top tips

■ **'Less is more when it comes to foundation, especially as we age.** I only apply base where I need it (on broken veins, under-eye shadows and the central T-zone) and leave the sides of my face make-up free, which prevents the foundation from looking like a mask.' Dayle Haddon, actress and model.

■ **Apply foundation in downward strokes.** This covers up pores well but avoids pushing pigment up and into them, which only serves to highlight them.

Look younger instantly

A useful rejuvenating tip is to change the type of foundation you use. All-over matte foundation may look good and feel more covering, but it can make skin look flat and lifeless; all-over sheen makes you look as though you're in your teens (ie, greasy). Look instantly modern and years younger with a natural skin glow that's dewy around the cheeks, temples and browbones, and matte along the T-zone. The latest formulations are sheer and lightweight, glide on the skin smoothly and evenly, yet cover well so you can play them up or down, depending on how good or bad your skin is.

concealer

There comes a point in all our lives when we lose that fresh clear bloom of youthful skin under the eyes, and exchange it for bluish, dark circles that tell us we've been overdoing it. Thank heavens for concealer!

what it does

High colour, dull skin, dark circles, thread veins or blemishes? Concealer is the best product to use to hide minor blemishes and even out tiny imperfections, and virtually every make-up artist agrees that if you only have time to apply one item of make-up, make it your concealer. 'When your skin looks perfect, you can get away with wearing nothing else at all,' says make-up artist Cheryl Phelps-Gardiner. The true art of make-up is learning how to conceal the things you don't want to see, and highlighting the bits you do. When matching the right concealer to your skin, choose a colour that is one shade lighter than your foundation. If it's too pale it will show up imperfections even more.

Highlighters are powders or creams for the face and eyes which contain shimmering micro-particles of titanium dioxide to catch the light and enhance natural 'highs' such as the browbones, cheeks and lips. However, by the very fact that they highlight, they should only be applied to flawless skin or else you'll show up everything.

what texture?

Concealers come in creams and lotions, sticks and wands. But ultimately it is the texture which is most important. Look for a creamy texture which is smooth to the touch, avoiding those which are greasy (and will slide off the area you are trying to cover) or too dry and chalky (which will collect on the skin in patches and highlight rather than conceal flaws.) Use a fine brush to apply concealer precisely where you want it, then continue with your usual base and powder.

how to apply

Under-eye concealers are lighter than those you'd use for spots and pimples. They often contain light-diffusing particles – the miracle ingredient for any woman over 30 – that bounce harsh light off and away from dark areas, making them appear brighter and a little more flawless.

For the best way to conceal dark circles, do as professional make-up artists do. Take the finest brush for precision, then pick up a tiny amount of concealer and blend it on the back of your hand. This way you end up with just a tiny amount on the brush, so you're less likely to overdo it. Now hold a mirror out in front of you at eye level, look ahead into it and put your chin down, while still looking into the mirror. This shows the darkness up at its worst. Now carefully paint the concealer only onto the dark areas (often in the innermost recessed corner of the eye). Pat into place with your index finger, lightly enough so that you don't actually remove any concealer, but sufficient to blend it in well. Finally, if it's quite a creamy concealer, apply a fine layer of translucent powder over the top to seal it in place.

If it's eye bags you want to conceal, always apply concealer on the area of shadow directly beneath the bag, not on it, otherwise you'll be highlighting rather than hiding it. Just prime your skin first with eye cream, leave it to absorb for as long as possible, then apply concealer before anything else.

which colour?

The best colour for a covering concealer is yellow-based, and remember, it should be only one or two shades lighter than your skin tone. The most common mistake is to choose a concealer which is too pale or too pink. These will just sit on your skin, rather than blend in seamlessly the way you need them to. You may have seen green concealer, designed to tone down redness, hide tiny red thread veins and high colour. This can look uneven and take on a greyish appearance when applied to the skin, so avoid using it unless you are very experienced in applying make-up. Other colour corrective concealers come in apricot, rose, white and lilac. They are designed to lift and brighten different types of complexions, but again, are best avoided by a novice.

which brush?

A concealer brush should be small but firm, and come to a point at the tip to enable precise application exactly where you want it. Make sure you keep the brush clean by washing it regularly, especially if you use it to camouflage spots and pimples. Your finger is a convenient way to apply concealer on the run; it often gives a light cover and makes it easy to blend away into the skin.

top tips

■ **If you want to cover up patches of redness** (such as around the nose or on the cheeks), use foundation rather than concealer. Concealer will highlight rather than hide the area you are trying to cover; foundation will blend in and appear less obvious.

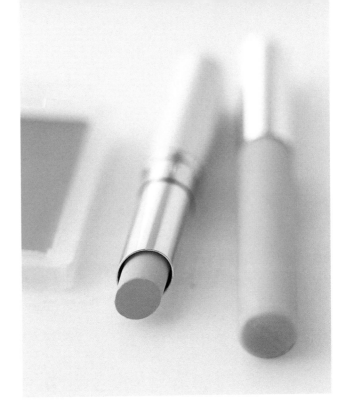

Make it last

The common mistake with daily make-up is that, although we may take time to touch up our lipstick or blusher during the course of the day, we rarely bother to add a little extra concealer, even though it's the most magical, age-defying make-up item we possess.

If you find your concealer slides off within a couple of hours, the chances are you didn't apply enough in the first place. Make-up artist Bobbi Brown recommends layering concealer when you want it to last. 'Apply two or three layers of concealer for best results and ensure that you powder over the top to keep it in place.' Bobbi also recommends applying a slightly brighter shade of blusher or lipstick than you might usually wear. This helps to draw attention away from your eyes and any darkness, especially if concealer has worn off.

powder

There was a time when every lady carried her face powder with her, and powdering one's face in public had an air of elegance about it. That era may be long gone, but powder remains one item of make-up you shouldn't be without.

what it does

Powder, purely and simply, absorbs excess shine. A super-fine translucent face powder can give skin an incredible softness, like looking through a camera lens that's steamed up. A girl's best friend if she has oily or combination skin (that is, oily down the T-zone), it is also easy to overdo and ultimately very ageing on skins over 35, as it can crack and cake. Powder has been less popular of late, with a shimmery, sexy skin sheen being more fashionable, especially in summer. But although this looks very fresh and pretty in magazine photographs, not everyone wants or suits a shiny face in real life. That's why powder will always be around.

what texture?

There is only one texture for face powder, and that's matte. The whole point is that you are removing any shine from your face. Don't confuse face powder with highlighting powders, which add a shimmer to skin. Other than that, you can choose from loose powder and pressed powder. Make-up artists generally prefer loose powder because it goes on in a lighter layer and tends to be super-fine in texture. Pressed powders come in a compact so they're great to carry around during the day for emergency touch-ups, but in general the powder tends to go on more heavily. Also handy to carry around are little books of blotting papers which contain several sheets of paper impregnated with a fine layer of powder.

how to apply

If you don't like to shine, pick up a little powder on a big brush or on a velour puff, dust off any excess, then dab a little powder down the centre of your face. Pay particular attention around the inner part of the eye, the nose, around the mouth and put a tiny amount on the forehead. Make sure you don't powder the cheeks and around the hairline. Powder is renowned for settling in the creases around the eyes and emphasising them even more. If you prefer to use pressed powder, pick up a little powder on a puff, dust off the excess on the back of your hand or a tissue, then press it into the areas of the skin you want to be matte. This gives a more lasting but slightly heavier finish than a brush, making it ideal for oily, Mediterranean skins. Never rub powder onto the skin: that is when it settles too heavily in the pores and the creases and looks unflattering.

which colour?

Translucent only. According to most make-up artists, while face powder is essential to keep the rest of your make-up in place and to blot out any shininess, it should be virtually invisible. Translucent powder is in effect colourless, which means that it won't interfere with the colour of your foundation or your blusher. However, some make-up artists prefer a yellow-toned powder, especially if your skin is more golden or olive, because it has a brightening effect, especially around dark circles.

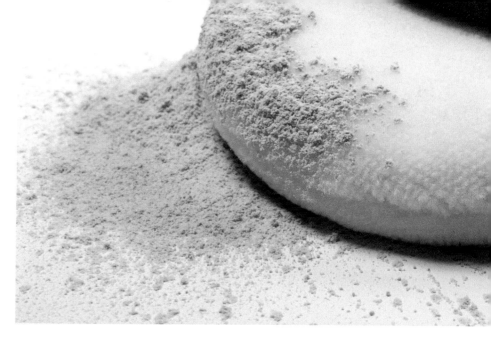

which brush?

A huge, soft powder brush that will sweep powder on and dust it off in a single movement is the best brush to use, especially if you have dry or mature skin, because it gives a softer finish. A velour powder puff is also useful for those who need a little extra powder to combat oiliness. A powder puff presses powder onto skin, so the finished effect is often a little heavier and best for younger skins, which tend to be oilier and less lined. Otherwise combine both: pat along the T-zone with a puff and lightly brush the cheeks.

top tips

■ **Check for excess.** When applying powder, always make sure that no particles have settled in your eyebrows or lashes. If they have, brush through immediately.

■ **Powder can go a little darker on the skin** when it is applied than it appears in the container, especially if the skin is greasy. If in doubt, always choose a slightly paler shade.

■ **When applying powder,** puff out your cheeks as you apply, to fill out any tiny lines around the mouth, and apply a very light dusting of loose powder.

■ **A fine layer of translucent powder** on the eyelids acts as a film between your skin and eye-shadow, so colour goes on more smoothly and evenly, and stays in place for longer.

■ **Combined two-in-one powder foundation** formulas are great for those who need to make up in a hurry, but make sure you use them lightly. They have a tendency to be quite covering, giving a heavier finish than you may actually want, and are often quite drying on more mature skins.

■ **If you need a matte finish,** but still find face powder too heavy or drying on the skin, use one of the latest gel cream make-up bases which contain tiny powder particles to stop the shine (such as those by No 7, Helena Rubinstein, Lancôme and Clinique). You can use them on clean skin along the T-zone under make-up, or on top of foundation to touch up shiny patches throughout the day. The trick is to pat and press them on to skin rather than wiping it on.

■ **Make-up on the mirror?** When carrying a pressed powder compact around in your bag, always try to keep the protective plastic cover over the powder. This will prevent your mirror from becoming powdery every time you want to use it.

blusher

As the most miraculous make-up item in your bag, don't just think of blusher as simply adding colour to your cheeks. Well-applied, it adds a wonderful glow to your whole face, enlivening your skin with a fresh, youthful radiance.

what it does

Every woman can benefit from the complexion-enhancing benefit of blusher, especially if you're a bit under the weather or have been burning the candle at both ends. You've probably heard the age-old advice to stop wearing black as you grow older: the reason for this is that our skin loses its natural pinky blush as it ages, so wearing black can make skin appear sallow and dull. However, blusher can help by adding an essential healthy glow. Lightly dusted over the cheekbones, chin and hairline, it adds youth, warmth and vitality in one easy step. 'Nothing makes a woman look prettier than blusher. It's the one item of make-up that can give skin a quick boost in the middle of the afternoon,' says Bobbi Brown.

what texture?

Most popular are the micro-fine powder blushers. Easy to apply and retouch, they allow you to add the lightest touch of colour to your face. Creams, which look attractive at first, have a tendency to be absorbed into dry skin, leaving creases. Gel blushers are tricky: they dry so quickly that they need an expert touch to avoid blotches. Look out for the latest powder cream formulations, which have a long-lasting semi-matte finish. However, they are a little heavier on colour than powders so you need a light hand. Fast becoming popular are 'multi-stick' blushers that vary from matte to semi-matte to shimmery, depending on the kind of look you like. These are great 'take it anywhere' make-up items simply because they don't spill, you apply them straight from the stick and blend onto your skin using your fingers, so you don't need a blusher brush in your bag either.

how to apply

Blusher should not be obvious. It should make you look like you're glowing from a country walk, or blushing from a kiss. It looks most youthful when dusted on the apple of the cheeks (their fullest, and so most youthful, part). Do as the models do: before applying blusher, they smile to push up the cheek muscles – a useful tip if your face lacks prominent cheekbones. Pick up a little colour on the brush and blow off the excess: on the back of the hand is often a convenient place to do it. Remember that it is easier to build up colour than take it away.

Dust over cheeks in a circular motion. Remember to carry the colour lightly round to the temples. 'Women often apply blusher looking full on into a mirror, forgetting that other people view their face from the sides too. Applying it this way will give a more natural look,' says Olivier Echaudemaison, Guerlain's make-up artist. Apply blusher to the brow bones to give warmth to the eyes, and across the brow close to the hairline to minimise a high forehead and gaunt temples. A touch on the chin softens a pointed or chiselled jawline. Never use blusher to shade and shape your face. It is there to add a bloom of fresh colour only.

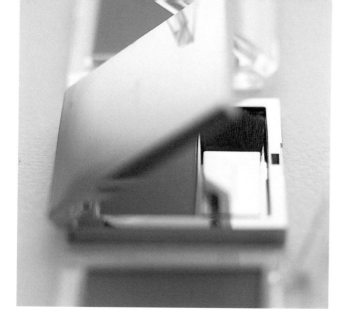

which colour?

Blusher looks unnatural if it doesn't tone well with your natural skin shade. Try to match it as closely as possible with the natural colour of your cheeks. As a rough guide: fair skins need sandy-pink; medium skins should opt for tawny-rose; yellow skins need fresh rose; and choose deep rose for dark skins.

Don't use bronzing powder as blusher unless your skin is medium to olive or dark, otherwise the effect tends to look rather muddy on the skin rather than fresh and pretty.

which brush?

Ideally, use a very soft, fat brush that follows the contours of your face and gives a softer veil of colour that blends well into your skin and makes it much easier to get the perfect application. Do try to avoid the tiny brushes that come in powder compacts – they are for emergencies only!

top tips

■ **If you overdo blusher,** use a damp cosmetic sponge to blend in a little more foundation, then dab on a little powder to blend.

■ **Can't see it?** Lightly retouch your cheekbones only. Don't be tempted to do a full re-application or you will probably end up overdoing it.

■ **Try this tip from Sophia Loren.** 'She always applies her blusher under her chin to soften her jawline and give her face an instant lift,' says Olivier Echaudemaison.

■ **'Blusher should always look as if your cheeks have been caught by the sun.** So apply colour on the cheekbones and not under them in the hollow, where it looks gaunt.' Make-up artist Mary Greenwell.

■ **Once you find the right shade** of blusher that adds a freshness to your skin, you'll never have to change the colour again, although you may vary the texture depending on the season and fashion.

■ **If you find that your choice of blusher just sits on your skin** and doesn't blend well, the shade is probably wrong. Go for a lighter, more neutral blush. You'll know when you get it right.

■ **If you have a full face,** place the blusher more towards your hairline and temples, and if you have very high cheekbones, place the blusher more towards your nose to give the effect of more rounded cheeks.

'nothing makes a woman look

prettier than blusher.

It's the one item of make-up that

can give skin a quick boost in the

middle of the afternoon.'

Bobbi Brown, make-up artist

mascara

Even if you never use any other item of make-up, mascara is the most indispensable beauty product for every woman. Just one coat and, in an instant, lashes look subtly defined. Add another coat and you'll look even more eye-catching.

what it does

Mascara thickens and emphasises your lashes, and rates as the most popular item of make-up for almost every woman. In fact, eyes look positively naked without it. Better still, you can even choose your mascara type – from lash-building products which contain filaments to thicken, to lash-lengthening types which often contain polymers for a natural, glossy finish, or water-resistant, long-lasting formulas.

what texture?

'A good mascara is one that stays looking glossy once it's dried,' says make-up artist Daniel Sandler. 'Dull lashes just don't look healthy.' The best new mascaras contain polymers which leave a sheer, even and often water-resistant coating on lashes. Another bonus is that polymers glide on top of each other, so that when you add a second coat it no longer clumps and drags on the first.

Lash-thickening mascaras contain water-attracting ingredients to moisturise and so swell lashes, plus polymers to seal in water and reduce stickiness, while lengthening mascaras contain film-forming molecules which give sheer, even cover, helping to define each lash from the root to the tip so they appear longer. New waterproof mascaras now contain volatile oils which instantly evaporate to leave a hard shiny coating to lashes, a little like nail polish. This makes them great in summer, but they need an oily remover to take off at the end of the day, so can seem a little harsh for day wear.

Fast becoming hugely popular once again since its heyday in the 1960s is block mascara: a solid cake of colour that is painted on with a small brush and gives a much denser finish to lashes. Make-up artists love block mascara and, because you paint it on, it's ideal for those with fair lashes who need to get the colour right onto the roots.

Research shows that eyelashes can become brittle and dry, as all hair can. If you find this is a problem, you may wish to use a lash primer or undercoat which conditions the lashes before applying mascara, makes them more flexible and often improves the application and wear as a result, too.

how to apply

Wipe the wand with a tissue because if the first coat is too heavy, lashes will stick together. Brush the upper lashes downwards from the top, and the lower lashes upwards from underneath. And apply sparingly: it's easy to overdo it on the first coat and then lashes look caked, stuck together and totally false. Finish by brushing through any lumps with a mascara comb, preferably metal, to separate lashes.

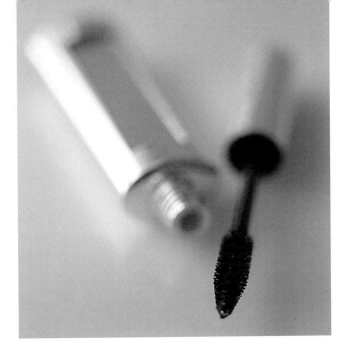

which colour?

If in doubt about which colour mascara will best suit you, stick to black or a brownish black. Coloured mascaras may be the height of fashion on the catwalks, but in real life they very rarely look flattering. Brown mascara gives lashes a hint of definition and suits those who like natural looking make-up. It is also the perfect colour for those with red hair or blonde lashes, for whom black mascara will be too harsh.

which brush?

As with all types of make-up brushes, mascara brushes come in a variety of styles, and each particular type can make a difference to the finished effect. Graduated bristles suit longer lashes and give a spiky finished look; curved bristles coat all the lashes at once, but often miss the roots; straight and slim bristles are great for applying mascara to those hard-to-reach lashes; spiral bristles are good for short or fine lashes and don't overload them; and hollow-fibre bristles hold lots of colour so that you get a thicker application for more volume.

top tips

■ **Always comb mascara through with an eyelash comb.** Choose one with metal teeth rather than plastic (see pages 114–15).

■ **To prevent clumpy lashes,** wipe your mascara brush with a tissue before you use it. You're not wasting any of it: if you wipe the brush on the side of the tube, it will clump even more quickly.

■ **If you have pale lashes** and can't reach the lash base with your mascara wand, use liquid eyeliner in a matching shade to paint on the bits you've missed.

■ **If you want to use an eyelash curler** to make lashes appear thicker and longer, curl your lashes before applying mascara otherwise the curler will cling to the mascara and pull the lashes.

■ **If your lashes are fine or sparse,** try smudging a little black eye pencil inside the lash line to create the illusion of thicker, darker lashes.

■ **If you smudge your mascara (or eyeshadow),** dip a cotton bud into a little eye make-up remover lotion and lightly dab the smear away.

Curl 'em

If you have straight lashes, you may find curling helps to add emphasis and give the illusion of bigger, wide-open eyes. To curl your lashes, look straight ahead into a mirror, position the curlers around the upper lashes, press down firmly and hold for a count of five. Then roll the curler up and away while holding the lashes, and repeat on the other eye.

eye-shadow

We rarely use eye-shadow to its full potential. You can't change the shape of your eyes, but with eye-shadow you can create the illusion of bigger, wider, narrower or deeper eyes with just a little clever shading and contouring.

what texture?

Eye-shadow is great for changing your look, both in terms of the colours and products you choose and the different ways in which you can apply them. If you're feeling in the middle of a make-up rut, now's the time to experiment. For the most modern look to your eye make-up, keep it simple. A clean sweep of a single colour, matte or shimmery, is just about all you need for a basic daytime look. Then experiment a little more for evening, using shadows to shape your eyes for more definition. Remember that matte eye-shadows are best for contouring, while iridescent shadows work as highlighters. Use dark shadows to create depth and to make prominent areas recede, and light shadows to emphasise and bring out other eye features.

how to apply

For longer lasting, crease-proof eye-shadow, it's important to prime your skin properly beforehand with an application of sheer, translucent face powder. Avoid putting eye cream on just beforehand or shadow will crease in seconds. Allow about 15 minutes for it to fully absorb. Smooth out your skin tone and cover any bluish veins with foundation, then use a velour powder puff and pat the eyelids with face powder.

Then get a matte eye-shadow that perfectly matches your skin tone and blend across the entire eyelid, from lashes to brow, using a shadow brush. Now you are in the perfect position to apply any shade of powder eye-shadow you choose. It will blend beautifully in a wash of colour that you can build up for more intensity, or to contour, and will stay in place longer. 'Always prime the eyelids with an undercoat of foundation and powder. You can shape and contour from this simple canvas,' says make-up artist Maggie Hunt.

■ **If your eyes are close-set,** concentrate light colours on the inner corners and darker shades on the outer edges of your eyes.

■ **If your eyes are wide-set,** do the opposite: dark shadow on the inner corners and light shadow on the outer corners.

■ **To lift droopy lids,** shade the outer corners of the eyes, tapering colour upwards and outwards.

■ **For longer lasting shadow,** apply powder eye-shadow with a damp brush. The shadow will dry into the skin as you blend it, and because it clings to the wet brush you'll avoid the problem of dry eye-shadow crumbling on to your cheek below, too.

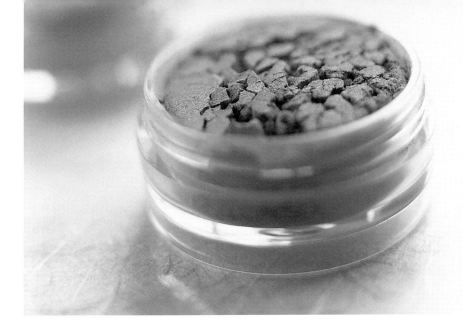

which colour?

As a rule, avoid matching your eye-shadow to the colour of your eyes, especially if your eyes are green or blue. If in doubt, neutral colours that contrast with your eye colour work best.

■ **If you have blonde hair:** with blue/grey eyes, wear taupe eye-shadow over the eyelids and brown to contour; with brown eyes, wear green over lids and a deeper green to contour; with green eyes, wear grey/blue over lids and grey to contour.

■ **If you have red hair:** with blue/grey eyes, wear peach eye-shadow over lids and mid brown to contour; with brown eyes, wear grey/green over lids and heather to contour; and with green eyes, wear lilac over lids and blue to contour.

■ **If you have brown/black hair:** with blue/grey eyes, lilac eye-shadow over the eyelids and heather to contour; with brown eyes, pale grey over lids and a slate grey to contour; with green eyes, wear pale lilac over lids and blue/grey to contour.

■ **If you have grey hair:** with blue/grey eyes, wear taupe eye-shadow over the eyelids and heather to contour; with brown eyes, wear lilac over the lids and heather to contour; with green eyes, wear pale blue over the lids and charcoal grey to contour.

which brush?

The best eye-shadow brush has short bristles that hold powder well, making colour easier to control and blend into the skin. If you use a creamy eye-shadow, fingers are best for blending. Avoid using the tiny sponge-tipped applicators that come with eye-shadow compacts. They are often hard to control and colour invariably goes on too heavily.

top tips

■ **To enhance small eyes,** avoid dark shadow and concentrate shading colour on the socket lines and outer edges. White pencil along the inner lower lid will also make the whites of the eye look bigger and brighter.

■ **To avoid eye-shadow falling on your skin,** apply a heavy dusting of loose powder on your cheek. It will catch any falling debris and you can then brush it away, leaving your make-up intact.

■ **If you want to use shimmer,** keep it subtle. It's worth remembering that shiny textures highlight imperfections. If you have mature skin, be cautious, but don't avoid them altogether. Always aim to place shimmer on areas where the skin is smooth such as the browbones.

eyeliner

Eyeliner gives eyes definition, gains attention from complete strangers, and becomes almost indispensable with age as lashes become sparse and eyes deeper set. Yet it is the one item of make-up that women find most difficult to control.

what texture?

If you're looking for a softer, subtle smoky eye that doesn't look harsh and obvious, choose a kohl eyeliner pencil. Especially good for those who are wary of eyeliner and always want to take it off the moment they've applied it, you can build up the line gradually and blend it softly away if it starts to look heavy.

Liquid eyeliner takes quite a bit of practise, but the overall effect is much more dramatic than with pencils. However, because it gives a very definite line, it can look a little harsh on older skin and tends to look more flattering on younger eyes which are smoother and less crepey.

how to apply

The best way to apply pencil liner is one third of the way along from the inner corner of the eye close to the lashes, tapering up and off at the corners. Then smudge-blend to get the degree of depth you want. For a really subtle eyeliner application, pull back the eyelid a little and fill in between the lashes from underneath.

The trick to applying perfect liquid eyeliner is with a steady hand: look down into a mirror lying flat on a table in front of you. This way you can see the whole eyelid, revealing exactly what you're doing. And it means you've got both hands free and can rest your elbow on the table to steady your hand. If the finished effect looks too harsh, you can soften it by adding a line of powder shadow over the top. Powder shadow worn as eyeliner gives the softest effect of all. To apply, pick up a little colour on an eye-shadow brush, dust off the excess on a tissue or the back of your hand, and blend close to the lashes on the upper and lower lids. If liner smears or blobs, dip a cotton bud in a little eye make-up remover lotion and carefully stroke away the mark. Powder and blend again. Now you should be able to finish where you left off.

The trend for wearing eyeliner inside the lower rim of the eyes goes in and out of fashion year after year, but one thing remains constant: ophthalmologists advise against it. Applying liner inside the eye may well enhance the overall look of your make-up (black gives a sexy, smoky, intense look while white is used to brighten the whites of the eyes on stage, making them appear bigger and wide-eyed), but it can also lead to irritation and even infection.

which colour?

Try shades other than black, too. If you have blue eyes, brown, navy or charcoal eyeliner looks softer and prettier than black. If you have brown eyes, then a deep brown looks more subtle; and if you have green eyes, try a brown or charcoal eyeliner.

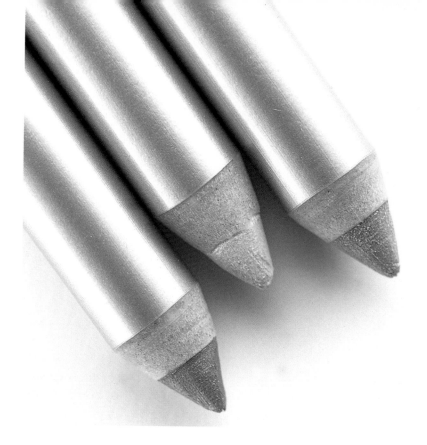

which brush?

Unless you are applying pencil eyeliner, a small, thin, fine-tipped brush that is gently rounded to a point for more precision makes the best eyeliner brush for liquid or cake eyeliner. If you are using kohl or pencil eyeliner, keep a few cotton buds in your make-up bag to blend and soften the line.

top tips

■ **If eyeliner makes your eyes look smaller,** add white kohl pencil on the inner rim of your eye. It's a theatrical trick that gives the illusion of bigger whites of the eyes.

■ **If your pencil liner rubs off too quickly,** try painting liquid liner underneath first. Then draw over the top with pencil and smudge-blend to get the softness. This also gives the pencil something to cling to, making it last longer.

■ **If the point of your eye pencil breaks off** while you're sharpening it, it means that the pencil is too soft. Put it in the fridge for an hour or two before sharpening so it'll be harder and less likely to break.

■ **'Always apply pencil liner across the entire eyelid** next to the lashes, tapering up and off at the corners,' says Jillian Veran of Bobbi Brown. 'Your eye doesn't start halfway across so why should your liner?'

■ **Practise makes perfect.** If you always seem to get a wobbly line, keep your elbows steady on a table, look down into a mirror laid flat, and stretch the skin along the lid before applying, so you have a smoother surface on which to draw your line.

eyebrows

Eyebrows are the most underrated part of your face. They influence the balance, feel and character of a face far more than any other single feature and can make a huge difference to the way you look.

why they matter

The arch, shape and width of your brows determine the expression on your face. If you make up your eyes but neglect your brows, your face will look 'unfinished', yet with the right shaping and products they can make you look bright-eyed and 10 years younger.

what texture?

Eyebrow pencils are firmer and more waxy than eye-shadow pencils, making them less likely to smudge, and enabling you to draw in brow hairs where you need to fill in. Brow powder gives a softer finish and is easy to use if you are learning how to emphasise your brows.

how to apply

Neat brows open up your eyes and enhance their shape. If eyebrows are shaped to balance the rest of the face, your eyes will automatically appear bigger. To get the shape of your brows right, hold a pencil along the side of your nose. The brow's inner edge should start vertically above the inner corner of the eye. Now lay the pencil from the outside edge of your nostril past the outer corner of your eye, and where it touches is where the brow should end (brows that stretch too far pull your eyes down, making them look droopy).

The arch of your brow should be about halfway along, just beyond the outer edge of the iris. If you are still unsure where exactly to pluck, check the shape before you begin by drawing over the hairs you want to pluck with a white pencil – it saves mistakes later. Bear in mind that a new shape is high maintenance and may need weekly or bi-weekly touch-ups.

If your brows are unruly, make sure they are well-groomed and try a clear eyebrow gel to keep hairs in place. Don't be too tempted to snip off the straggly tops of brows: it does make brows look sharper, but it's easy to make mistakes, so leave it to the professionals.

which colour?

The number one rule is 'don't overdo brow colour'. Over-defined brows which are too dark in colour will only make you look like a clown. Always keep colours soft and suitable for your colouring. If your brows are pale, thin or sparse, fill in with a brow pencil that matches the natural colour of your brows or is a tone lighter than them. Groom them so they follow the shape of your eyes.

If you don't know where to start, try drawing the shape you want with a pencil and use it as a guide for applying colour. Keep the colour light to complement your hair. Using a brow pencil, draw colour in with tiny, upward feathery strokes in the direction of hair growth, and subtly extend the line at the outer corners. Then blend with a stiff brow brush, working the colour through the brows upwards and outwards, following the shape of the natural browline.

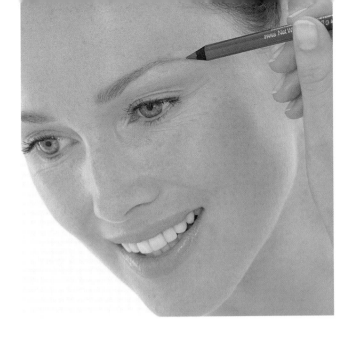

If you've over-plucked your eyebrows over the years and your brows are now too thin, try to grow them back and use a mushroom powder shadow to enhance them. Decide which areas need filling in with pencil and resist the urge to pluck any new hairs growing through. Apply colour to the arch first, then go back to the inner edge and taper off to the end. By using this method you won't end up with a heavy-looking brow which is hard to remedy afterwards.

which tweezers and brush?

Metal tweezers with an angled head and fine tip are the easiest to use for plucking eyebrows, whether you are just tidying the brows or creating a definite shape. When applying colour to the eyebrows, use a stiff brow brush for thorough blending.

top tips

■ **If you find plucking too painful,** ice your brows before plucking to numb the pain, or try a little baby teething gel which contains an anaesthetic. Tea tree oil will reduce any irritation if some of the plucked hairs were a little coarse.

■ **If your brows are too thick** and you simply don't know where to start, have a professional brow-shaping session in a salon. Once you have the desired shape, it's easier to maintain yourself.

■ **Soap is an excellent brow tamer.** If you have hairs that simply insist on lying in an awkward direction, rub a clean mascara brush on a wet bar of soap and brush unruly brow hairs into place.

■ **If you like wearing shimmery highlighter on the browbone,** it is important to pluck the hairs in this area or stray hairs will be highlighted and look extremely unflattering. Adding a smear of shimmery pale powder to the eyebrows prior to plucking is a useful way to emphasize which hairs you need to remove.

How to pluck

Take your time and ideally use a magnifying mirror in daylight when plucking your eyebrows. Always pluck one hair at a time from underneath the natural brow line. Never shape the top hairs or they will end up patchy and unbalanced. Pull each hair out with a swift, sharp tug in the direction it is growing, holding the skin taut with the other hand as you pull. Plucking after a shower or bath is often less painful because skin is softer.

Comb brows into shape, then take a good look at where you want to pluck. Start by tidying up obvious stray hairs – this may be all you need to make a difference. For a more definite shape, keep using the pencil as your rule. As you pluck, step back and make sure each brow matches the other: do a few hairs on one side then some on the other so they balance.

lipstick

Lipstick is one of the most essential items of a woman's make-up, and even those of us who rarely use face powders or lotions may feel bare and uncomfortable without a lipstick to hand in the bottom of the bag.

what lipsticks should do

Most lipsticks consist of a fatty base to ensure that the product stays firm but is easily spread, and colour is added by dyes or pigments. A good lipstick must be soft enough to adhere to the lips smoothly and should stay there when we eat, drink and kiss the evening away. However as every wearer knows, it takes a dry lipstick indeed to stay in place, and the majority of cosmetics manufacturers are obsessed with finding the ultimate lipstick that lasts without drying the lips.

what texture?

Everything goes sheer and shimmery in summer to reflect the warmth of the sun, lighter layers and the overall mood. Come winter however, you can guarantee that everything becomes deeper, richer, more matte and more defined, to go with heavier fabrics and darker hues.

But ultimately it's what you like that matters. So if you like gloss, but are over 50, you can still wear it, but place it on the centre of the bottom lip where it looks more sophisticated and far more flattering than all over. If you have thin lips, try a coloured lip balm or a shimmery shade which enhances them and make lips look groomed, rather than drawing a line around them to make them look bigger artificially.

■ **Gloss** (otherwise known as lip shine, lip lacquer, polish or shimmer) gives lips a softer, more youthful look, and keeps them feeling smoother than traditional lipstick. Better still, you don't even have to invest in a new one: simply buy a clear gloss or a pot of Vaseline, and apply over the top of your all-time favourite lip colour to get the effect. The way to wear it is as a highlighter to enhance your mouth's natural colour. Dab on the centre of the top and bottom lips, press lips together and you'll get the illusion of all-over gloss without the slip factor.

■ **Matte** delivers the drama of colour without the distracting shine of cream or gloss. But as a result it is often as dry as the Sahara and may leave lips feeling taut and dry within hours. That's because matte lipsticks contain a high percentage of powder and, although this is what makes them long-lasting, you might find you want something a little less flat. If you have a matte lip colour you like, but still find it drying, mix it with a little lip balm. It won't last quite as long as if you use it on its own, but your lips will certainly feel more comfortable.

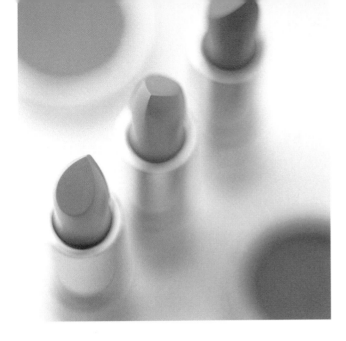

The latest breed in long-lasting (or 'transfer-resistant') lip colours uses polymers and silicones in an attempt to remove the dryness, yet still enable the colour to stay in place for hours. If, however you do like the effect of matte lip colour, just remember that matte is ageing, dark flat shades can look harsh next to the complexion, and it makes lips look smaller, because it doesn't reflect the light.

■ **Creamy, satin, demi-matte lip colours** give a softer finish than matte, but are infinitely more sophisticated than gloss. They are for those who want rich texture but don't want to compromise on colour. Best of all, they make dark shades appear softer, prettier and more flattering. The best way to apply creamy formulas is to blot them with a tissue, powder on top, then re-apply with a lip brush, because they have a greater tendency to smear. This way, the first coat stains your lips a little, and then helps the second coat stay in place better.

■ **Lip-liner** Outlining your lips gives them the stronger definition they may need, especially as they lose their natural plumpness and colour with age. The firm texture of a good lip pencil also enables you to touch up an uneven outline and helps to prevent lipstick from bleeding into any surrounding fine lines or wrinkles. For a longer lasting finish, you can also apply pencil in place of lipstick to colour in the entire lip area – use the side of the pencil to fill in. Then soften with a coat of lip balm, which prevents your lips from drying out and gives a more modern sheen, rather than flat matte colour which looks hard.

If you have yet to try lip pencils, or find them difficult to use, it will help to practise creating a lip line that doesn't look artificial or uneven. If in doubt, always choose a neutral lip pencil which matches your lip tone, so it gives a more subtle finish. Start by tracing the pencil along the actual lip line itself. Try to avoid drawing outside your natural lip line, otherwise you'll end up with a very unattractive rim around your mouth once the lip colour wears off. At the very most, make-up artists recommend drawing next to your actual line – either outside to make them look fuller, or inside to make them look thinner. Then, to make a pencilled mouth look less crisp, they run a dry brush around the edge to soften the line.

'husbands don't like their wives wearing red lipstick; it's too sexy and gets her noticed. I say wear it.'

Olivier Echaudemaison, make-up artist at Guerlain

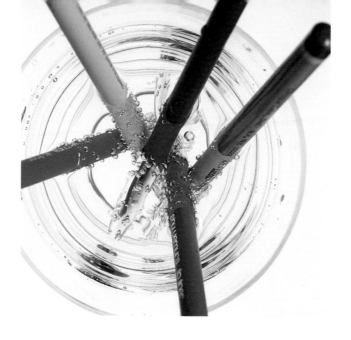

how to apply

Just how well your lipstick goes on and stays on has a lot to do with the way you prime your lips beforehand. Dry, dehydrated lips invariably soak up emollients, leaving behind an uneven stain, whereas an overly moist mouth means that even the longest lasting formula will slide off in seconds because it has nothing to cling to. Lip primers condition lips while giving colour something to cling to. It's an extra step in your regime, but might be worth the effort if you find your lipstick disappears fast.

To ensure the very best application, first prepare your lips with a smear of moisturising lip balm. Apply over your lips at the beginning of your make-up, and leave to absorb while you do your face and eyes. After finishing the rest of the face, blot off any excess balm that hasn't been absorbed with a tissue. The result? Lips look absolutely smooth, but not so slick that colour slides right off them.

which colour?

Choosing the lip colour to suit your complexion isn't easy. First you obviously have to think about the kind of look you want to create, whether it's a dark, dramatic mouth, a pretty pastel pinky mouth or a natural 'barely there at all' mouth. We can all wear a selection these days to change the way we look instantly, but the trick is to achieve a balance whereby they always flatter you.

how to choose?

First hold a lip colour up near your face and see if its tone complements your hair and skin colour. For hygiene, never test a lip colour straight from a tube onto your mouth. The next best place is on the pad of your fingertip. Skin here is more pinky and similar to the colour of your lips.

Now you can experiment. Here are a few basic colour theories. While deep, rich colours warm the complexion, pale colours drain it. Therefore, if you choose a colour somewhere between the two for a daytime shade, your job is instantly made easier. Pinky-brown shades which closely match your actual lip colour suit almost everyone and give the most natural look. Brown and toffee tones are flattering too, offering subtle definition without being garish. The popularity of red comes and goes, but it's a classic, chic colour. It's a bold statement, needs precise application and a certain amount of confidence to carry it off. And reds can be hard on fair skin. Either go for the dramatic contrast or wear it in softer berry shades. Few people can wear blue-toned reds and pinks, which invariably look harsh on fair or older skins, so if in doubt go for golden, yellow-toned colours which illuminate the skin.

which brush?

You can apply lip colour straight from the bullet, with a wand or with your fingertips, but none of these methods give you the control and accuracy of a lip brush. Professional make-up artists wouldn't be without theirs. It allows you to spread colour more evenly over the lips, enables colour to stay on that bit longer, and because you don't overload your lips with colour you inevitably use up less lipstick, so it's cheaper in the long run. In addition, it gives a softer look to lip liner, because you can blend away any harsh, obvious edges. Every make-up bag should carry a retractable lip brush – one that has its own case so it's easier to carry around and stays cleaner, and more hygienic. Otherwise look for a slim, flat brush with flexible bristles that should be about 8mm: neither too long to control, nor too short to be hard and inflexible.

top tips

■ **If you have fine lines around your mouth,** make sure that you carry your usual moisturiser over your lips as part of your daily skincare regime. Lip primers have conditioning formulas to provide a no-bleed base for lipstick, yet protect your lips from becoming dry. Use a lip pencil to accentuate your natural lip line and to hold colour in place through the day.

■ **If your lips are dry or cracked,** protect them with lip balm containing an SPF15. Re-apply the balm as often as you can remember throughout the day. Don't wait for them to get dry.

■ **If you suffer from cold sores,** you should use a sunscreen on your lips of no less than SPF15. The sun stimulates the herpes virus, but with adequate protection you should find you suffer far less.

■ **For a DIY conditioning lip mask,** give your lips a coat of vitamin E oil. Mix 5ml of oil with one drop of rose oil. It gives lips an instant natural shine without colour and helps to condition and protect their sensitive skin. Apply at night and never under lipstick – oils will make colour slide off in seconds.

Lipstick shapes

After a few applications your lipstick bullet starts to take on a whole new shape and meaning. First, it clearly indicates the way you apply your lipstick, but it may even reveal a certain side to your character.

■ **Flat shaped** This suggests that you apply lipstick to the bottom lip only and then press your lips together to coat both of them. It intimates that you're matter-of-fact, like to do things on the spot and swiftly, and have a no-nonsense kind of approach.

■ **Sloping** A lipstick that is flat on one side and pointing upwards on the other suggests that you apply it at an angle with your bottom lip open. You're likely to be sexy, seek attention and usually get it, but can be quite stressed. Psychologists say that the steeper the slope, the greater the stress.

■ **Pointy** When the lipstick is shaped a bit like the roof of a house – low at the sides and rising to a point in the middle – the chances are you apply your lipstick evenly to both top and bottom lips. Psychologically speaking you have a calm, balanced and neat personality.

■ **Bullet** If your lipstick becomes completely dome-like in shape, it means that, even without realising it, you are evenly sculpting the shape of your lipstick much as you would an ice cream cone. This indicates that you have a thoughtful, quiet but very smart personality.

the best tools for the job

■ **Eye-shadow brush:** a small, short brush, cut full and square, which enables you to pick up just the right amount of powder eye-shadow, creating a clean sweep of colour that's easy to blend.

■ **Eyeliner brush:** a small, thin, fine-tipped brush which is gently rounded to a point to create a more precise line next to, and between, the lashes. Use this brush damp, with either a cake eyeliner (a solid block of colour) or powder eye-shadow.

■ **Eyebrow brush:** needs to be short and firm, with coarse bristles clipped at an angle to follow the natural curve of the brow more easily. This allows for a cleaner, more even application of powder shadow along the brows.

■ **Metal slanted tweezers:** these are angled and pointed, and rarely miss a single hair. Be careful when handling them, though: if you drop metal tweezers they can quickly become blunt.

■ **Concealer brush:** a finely pointed, small brush with soft but short controllable bristles which are designed to accurately 'paint out' minor blemishes.

■ **Metal eyelash comb:** designed to remove any clumps of mascara and comb through lashes so they separate perfectly. The only ones worth choosing and using have metal teeth.

■ **Blusher brush:** a soft, rounded brush with gently tapered sides which help to contour and sculpt the cheeks without leaving stripes of colour.

■ **Powder brush:** a large, soft-bristled brush which sweeps over the entire face and neck without leaving an obvious layer of powder. Make-up artists much prefer using a big brush to a velour puff, especially on more mature skins, as the effect is softer and more flattering.

■ **Lipbrush:** a small brush with short controllable bristles – much like a concealer brush, but tapered to a square, flat tip. This shape makes it easier to outline and define the contour of the lips without leaving the kind of obvious rim you get with a lip pencil.

■ **Metal eyelash curlers:** to curl straight lashes or to help the odd stray eyelash curl up neatly with the rest. Curling instantly wakes up the eyes, giving them a more youthful appearance.

■ **Make-up brushes made from real hair,** such as sable and goat, last longer and feel softer and more luxurious on the skin than synthetic bristles; but they are also far more expensive.

■ **When it comes to powder and blusher,** the softer the brush, the softer the finish to your make-up. However, if you doubt how much use you'll get out of each brush, buy a cheaper option for eye-shadow, liner, lip and brow brushes, and splash out on the brushes for your base.

■ **Clean make-up brushes regularly,** every week, in mild soapy water to prevent a build-up of bacteria. Don't be tempted to skip this process.

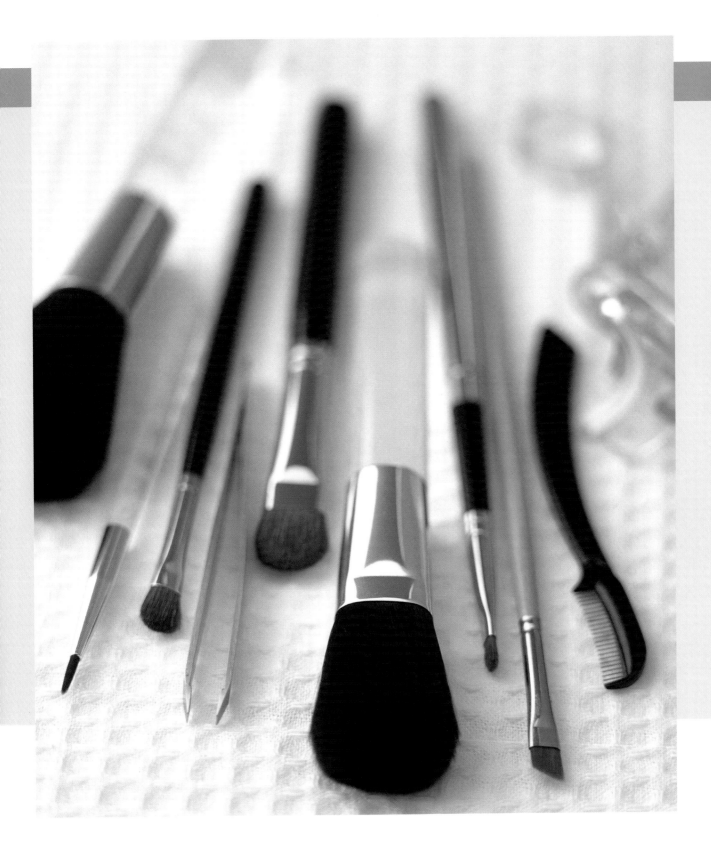

specialist make-up

Clever tricks to brighten you up and tone you down.

■ **Colour corrective lotions or powders** work by counterbalancing their opposite hue, toning down or brightening the complexion and helping to minimise imperfections. If you want to try a colour corrective product, the key is in making it work with your existing make-up rather than letting it sit on your skin in a separate layer. Blend your chosen colour with your usual powder or foundation, then apply to clean skin, for a subte, flattering effect.

Green takes the redness out of spots and blemishes, red thread veins, ruddy cheeks and sunburn. However, red and green make grey. Use the tiniest amount, otherwise your skin will take on a greyish tinge. Apricot is a great radiance booster and pick-me-up for tired dull skin. Lilac revives tired, sallow skin and adds radiance under harsh lights. Yellow evens out skin tone and can be mixed with foundation or used as a powder, to give the complexion a flattering finish. Blue works with pale skin, giving it an ethereal quality, while white adds luminosity and lightens dark circles under the eyes.

Always take great care when using these coloured products. If you apply too much green, for instance, skin soon looks greyish; use too much lilac and skin looks washed out.

■ **Tinted moisturiser** creates the perfect balance between skincare and make-up. Ideal in spring, when your skin needs more moisture after the cold winter, yet you want to add a bit of healthy radiant colour, these creams are quite sheer and blend in easily with the skin to boost your natural skin tone.

■ **Bronzing powder** Come summer, many of us eagerly swap blusher for bronzing powder in order to achieve a more golden, sun-kissed look. However, it does not take much for bronzers to turn you quickly from a delicate rose into a disco diva. If you like bronzing powder and want to master the art of making it look natural rather than muddy, apply it on top of powder.

'A lot of women apply bronzing powder straight on top of moisturiser,' says make-up artist John Gustafson. 'But then it sticks, looks heavy and just goes completely wrong. You need to put a neutral powder underneath for a really natural finish, then think about where the sun usually hits your face – across the bridge of the nose, tops of cheeks, and brow bones – and only use it there. Bronze becomes universally wearable when it's golden brown, not coppery. Pick a bronzer that brightens your skin to the shade you'd naturally turn after being in the sun.'

■ **False lashes** are strictly for high drama effects, if only because they can be so tricky to apply and few of us have the confidence to wear them without imagining them crawling down our cheeks halfway through the evening. Model Naomi Campbell is famous for wearing false lashes, day and night. 'I like wearing a few individual lashes to make my lashes look thicker and more eye-catching,' says make-up artist Cheryl Phelps-Gardiner.

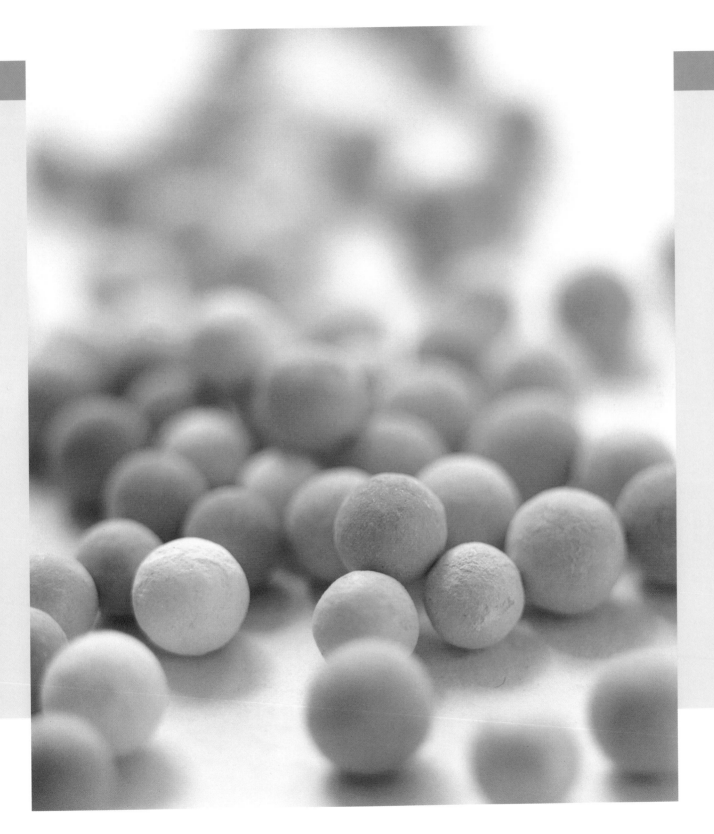

how to find your perfect colours

Make-up invariably works best when it complements your eyes, hair colour and skin tone. Review your make-up colours on a regular basis, and by becoming more in tune with your looks you'll quickly learn what suits you best.

brunettes

The colours that suit brunettes vary considerably from person to person. While some have cool-toned skin with perhaps grey eyes, others have warmer, golden skin. The shades that will best enhance your eyes also vary greatly depending on your eye colour.

■ **Light/medium brown hair** To decide whether you need warm rather than cool colours, be guided by whether or not your hair has any red or golden lights in it, and whether your skin has a yellow undertone. If your skin is pale, and you have blue or green eyes and no warm highlights in your hair, stick to cool colours such as lilac, lavender, aquas, taupe and cool browns on your eyes. Cool pinks and pale plums will define the cheeks and complement your cool skin tone. Pinky brown, fuchsia, heather, plums and a true red make the perfect lipstick collection.

■ **Rich brown hair** Olive skin and dark brown eyes are easy for matching colours. Bronze, taupe, deep browns, warm olive greens and rich charcoal give extra definition to your eyes. Terracotta and tawny blusher suits your yellow-based skin tone; while toffee, cinnamon and browny reds work on the lips.

blondes

From a platinum blonde with pale skin and light eyes to a golden honey-toned blonde with green eyes, or an olive-skinned blonde with deep brown eyes, the colours that suit you will vary immensely.

■ **Ash blondes/grey hair** If you have pale skin and blue or green eyes, cool-toned make-up will suit you best. For example, red lipsticks should be blue-reds, such as burgundy, rather than hot orangey reds. Pale eyes come to life when you use a dark contrasting colour eye-shadow such as charcoal, deep lavender, brown or navy. Pale greys, silver, beige and pastels also work well with white-blonde hair. Cool pink, plum and rose-beige blushers will give a natural flush to the cheeks, and mauve, wine, berry, soft fuchsia and cappuccino brown make great lip colours.

■ **Golden blondes** All your colours should ideally have a warmth to them, such as honey brown, bronze and gold. Ivory, champagne and gold are pretty for the eyes too. Warm pinks, peach and corals look good on your cheeks, and can also be used on lips, along with apricot, peachy browns and soft reds.

■ **Rich blondes** Go for brown-based shades such as gold, champagne, golden brown and khakis for the eyes. For cheeks, choose peaches and tawny browns. You can get away with both pale and deep shades of lip colour. Peach with a hint of brown and browny reds are ideal.

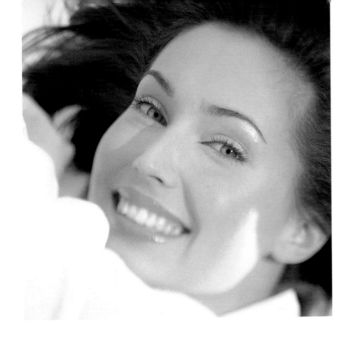
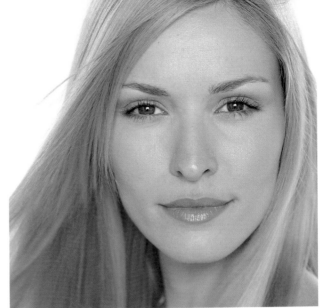

redheads

Generally speaking, redheads look best in warm rather than cool colours, which complement the warmth in the hair. However you may find that occasionally shades with a hint of blue in them create an exciting contrast to red. Predictably, make-up artists choose amber and spicy shades for redheads, but from time to time, for a change, a vibrant pink can look stunning.

■ **Pale red hair** If you have green or blue eyes, boost their colour with terracottas, golds and coppery browns. Peach, apricot and tawny brown blushers work well, while lip colours can range from cinnamon and brick to peachy brown and poppy red.

■ **Vibrant red/auburn hair** Your choice of eye-shadow will depend on the colour of your eyes. Blue and green eyes will be enhanced with the same shades as for pale redheads; but if you have brown eyes (and probably darker lashes and brows) you will suit beige, taupe, coffee, olive and bronze better. Warm chestnut and peachy brown blushers are a natural choice, while obvious lipstick choices are terracotta, peachy browns and berry tones.

Going grey?

As we age and our hair colour fades to grey or white, our skin also loses colour and, as a result, the make-up we wore in the past becomes too much for our new hair and skin colouring. However, it is a common mistake for women who have gone grey to feel that they need to wear brighter make-up to compensate. On the contrary, now's the time to focus on neutral and natural colours that are timeless.

Less really is more when it comes to choosing colours to suit grey hair and more mature skin tones. Use less eye-shadow than previously and find a selection of warm lip colours that work well for you. Warm your skin up with a soft coral or peach blusher, but keep everything else subtle and soft. For the best choice of colours to suit your complexion, choose eye-shadow that contrasts with the colour of your eyes. Stick to the same rules that apply to ash blondes (see opposite), and choose the softest shade and the softest texture available.

asian and black

Dark and black skins look good in a wide range of colours. Just make sure they complement each other: warm with warm, and cool with cool. Avoid any powders which contain too much white – these will simply look grey on black skin.

■ **Oriental** Your black hair and pale yet warm skin tone and dark eyes are often best defined by neutral shades on the eyes (such as ivory, taupe, coffee and beige) and deeper colours on the lips. Black eyeliner is virtually a must to lift the eyelids. Avoid dark eye-shadows which will make eyes seem smaller. For cheeks, opt for golden and tawny brown blusher, and go bold on the mouth with vibrant red, pinky browns, berry tones and spicy shades.

■ **Pale black skin** If you have warm golden or reddish tones in your hair, your brown eyes will look more striking with golden browns, copper and warm beige. Choose warm terracotta or chestnut blusher, and sheer browns, wines and burgundies for lips.

■ **Deep black skin** Your dark brown eyes, deep black skin and black hair can wear a vast range of colours, from purples and pinks to reds, golds and charcoal. The latter is your ideal choice for eyeliner, and works well with lilac, purple, silver, bronze and gold eye-shadows. Blusher can be anything from fuchsia to terracotta. Highlighter on the tops of the cheeks and brow bones is very flattering for evening. And for lips go for ruby reds, spicy shades, wine and berries, damson, terracotta, or simply a sheer, shimmery, sexy lip balm.

how to choose new make-up

■ **Beware of poor lighting in the store.** Go to a window and check make-up in daylight by a window before you decide to buy: colours often look very different on your skin in different lights.

■ **When choosing a new lip colour,** first hold it up near your face and see if its tone flatters your hair and skin colour, then try the colour out on the pad of your fingertip. The skin here is more pink than on the back of your hand and similar to the natural colour of your lips. Finally, if you think it's a good colour choice, use a cotton bud to apply a little on to your lips. Never test a lip colour straight from the tube onto your mouth.

■ **When choosing a new foundation,** test it along your jawline. This is where you need the colour to match perfectly. Apply stripes of four or five different shades next to each other. The perfect colour will be the one you cannot see sitting on your skin.

■ **When choosing a new eye-shadow,** first decide where you want to place the colour and whether it is to highlight (pale or shimmery tones) or shape and shade (dark and matte tones). Next, decide whether your natural skin tone is warm (golden, olive tones) or cool (fair, pinky tones) and opt for a shade that matches in warmth.

■ **Do seek advice from the make-up counter** in your favourite department store. The best advice generally comes from those make-up companies such as Bobbi Brown, Laura Mercier and MAC, who use fully trained make-up artists at the counter and believe in subtly accentuating a woman's good looks.

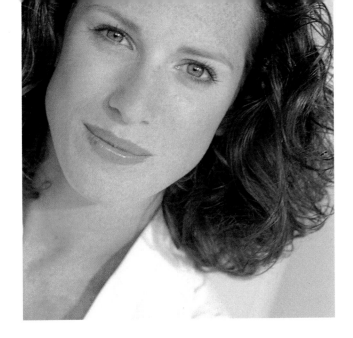

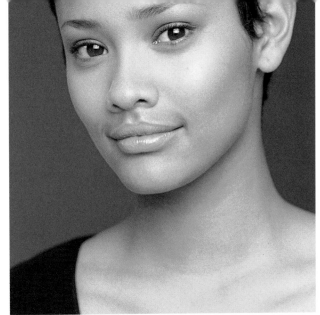

Your true colours

Who says redheads shouldn't wear red? Colour psychologists believe that the colours you wear can dramatically change the way you feel as much as the way you look.

■ **Blue** is universally liked as a colour. It is fresh, open, trusting and makes you feel confident and in control when you wear it.

■ **White** is deemed as pure, fresh, innocent and clean, and represents a new beginning. Wearing white will put you in a positive and forward-thinking mood, so it's a good choice if you are feeling under stress and need an optimistic approach to the day ahead.

■ **Green** means lush, verdant, young and fresh. In colour psychology it is a sign of inspiration, of growing mentally and bursting with new ideas. This is the colour to choose when you want time to think and be introspective, rather than when you are in the mood to get up and go.

■ **Red** is power, strength. The colour of energy and seduction. From a psychologist's point of view, if you wear red either you're very lively, or you'd like to be. Either way, red demands attention. It is an exciting, assertive, dynamic and passionate colour, but at the same time it is a rather good colour to hide behind, so choose it when you feel sluggish too, to give the impression of having more energy than you feel.

■ **Yellow** gives a bright, happy, sunny impression to those around you. It is an extrovert, positive and outward-looking colour and its brightness is believed to symbolise intelligence. So whenever you want to boost yourself out of a melancholic state of mind, wear yellow.

■ **Black** is associated with chic elegance, and women love wearing it because it is slimming. But black is not a colour, it's a statement. It says you are independent, unrestricted and rebellious. It allows you to behave in a way that might even be the opposite of how you really feel, so it's great for those times when you want to feel more assertive and individual than you really are.

eyes

Your eyes are the most expressive part of your face and the feature you'll most likely want to emphasise. Experiment with different colours and textures, and use make-up to shape your eyes and create different looks.

how to enhance eyes

A little make-up know-how can be rather handy when you want to play up your best features. However, most of us are not blessed with 'perfect' looks (make-up artists consider almond-shaped eyes as the ideal shape to make up) and sometimes we have to seek a little help from our cosmetics. This is where eye-shadow comes into its own.

While the prospect of shaping and shading your eyes may seem rather daunting at first, you only have to learn one basic rule and you'll be amazed at how easy it is to master. Simply remember that when it comes to eyes, it's all about shadow play. Use light and dark shadows to enhance and minimise. Play with the texture too, bearing in mind that shimmery shades accentuate by catching the light, while matte textures make everything look flatter.

small eyes

Apply a pale eye-shadow over the entire eyelid and up to the brow bone, then add a slightly darker colour in the socket line to emphasise the contour. Now place a dab of white eye-shadow on the brow bone to help open out the eyes even more.

large eyes

If you want to reduce an area, stick to dark, matte shades of eye-shadow. For large eyelids choose a deeper eye colour and apply over the lid and into the socket, then blend well.

wide-set eyes

Apply a pale shade of eye-shadow over the entire lid then add a deeper colour into and above the crease on the inner half of the eye only. Next, apply eyeliner all along the upper lid, making it slightly thicker at the inner corner of the eye.

close-set eyes

Apply pale shadow on the inner corners to widen, then blend dark shadow on the outer corner for emphasis. Apply eyeliner next, along the upper and lower lash line, winging it out at the sides.

Eye essentials

■ **'Eyelash curlers make your eyes look bigger,** make lashes look longer and give an instant lift to the face. Those by Shu Uemura are the best,' says make-up artist Roxanne New.

■ **'If you're not wearing much eye make-up,** wear navy mascara rather than black or brown,' says make-up artist Ariane Poole. 'It makes eyes look more vibrant and sparkling.'

■ **'If you have blonde eyelashes,** don't dye them,' says Maggie Hunt. 'Paint mascara on to the roots of the lashes using a fine eyeliner brush. It takes time but makes a huge difference.'

■ **Prime your eyelids first** for longer lasting, crease-proof eye-shadow by using a velour powder puff and patting the eyelids with a fine layer of face powder. This will enable different shades of eye-shadow to blend better together, so there are no obvious harsh edges left behind, and any shaping won't look too artificial.

■ **Experiment more with colour.** It's difficult to choose the ultimate brown eye-shadow that suits your particular pair of eyes when one cosmetics company alone may have over 50 different shades of brown to choose from. However, if you don't quite get the shade right when buying, try creating your own (as make-up artists do) by blending two different shades together. Powder shadows can be mixed on the back of your hand using a brush or just your fingertips.

■ **To enhance your eyes for going out in the evening,** add a tiny amount of pale, shimmery white or ice blue powder just on the inner corners of your eyes. It makes them shine, and is particularly effective if your eyes are close-set.

■ **For longer lasting finish,** apply powder eye-shadow with a damp brush. The powder will dry onto the skin as you blend it, and because it clings to the wet brush you'll avoid the problem of powder crumbling down on to your cheek.

cheeks

Just as you can shape your eyes to make them look larger, or closer-set, you can contour your cheeks to make your face look slimmer, fuller, longer or more rounded. The trick is to always keep it natural.

don't overdo it

The 70s trend for striping the face with bands of blusher, highlighter and shaper was possibly one of the worst make-up ideas ever. Who has the time, yet alone the inclination, to be that artificial with make-up? And the face is bound to look out of balance. Most make-up artists agree that shaping and shading the face is too tricky, and is strictly for the camera. 'The most important thing to remember is not to over-compensate,' believes Bobbi Brown. 'Use blusher to give your face a lift and to add a little colour, but don't waste your time trying to contour in chiselled cheekbones.'

how to apply blusher

According to Bobbi, blusher should always be applied on the apple of the cheek, which is where colour would naturally rise if you were embarrassed, exhausted or flushed. In this area it also makes the face look more youthful, especially once the face loses its plumpness and begins to hollow with age. 'To find the exact spot, smile in an exaggerated way. The apple is the round, lifted part of your face. And make sure you blend colour up into the hairline at the sides.'

However, if you have a round or wide face and your cheekbones are virtually non-existent, Roxanne New recommends placing colour on the cheekbones too, for a natural-looking way to create contours. 'Pick up the tiniest amount of blusher on the brush, dust off the excess and then, starting at the ears, make a semi-circular swoosh along the cheekbone, finishing on the apple of the cheek. Repeat a few times to build up the colour satisfactorily. Finally, wipe the brush, to remove as much of the colour as possible, and sweep the brush in the usual direction, from the apple to the ear, to soften the effect and ensure that fine facial hairs are lying flat.'

If you have a narrow face, you will probably benefit from a little shimmery highlighter placed along the top of the cheekbones to 'fill out'. Apply your blusher on the apples of the cheeks as usual to help give the impression of full cheeks, then apply a touch of sheer gloss along the tops of the cheekbones. Placed here it will widen. 'Using a shine stick, such as Nars Multiple, on upper cheekbones, the Cupid's bow of the lips and along the jawline, gives back the bloom and natural sheen of youth to older skins,' says Cheryl Phelps-Gardiner.

Cheek essentials

■ **'Whatever blusher you choose,** make sure it's slightly pink so skin stays looking baby fresh,' says make-up artist Daniel Sandler. 'Browny blusher tends to look muddy.'

■ **'If your blusher looks too bright,** soften it by layering a neutral blush colour over the top,' recommends Bobbi Brown.

■ **'Always apply blusher as the final step in your make-up,'** advises Maggie Hunt. 'The last thing you want to do is overplay its subtlety by applying too much colour.'

■ **Make-up professionals tend to use a matte brown powder** to contour and shape the face. If you want to do a little face shaping but are wary of using any product that looks too heavy, Maggie Hunt suggests using bronzing powder instead, especially around the chin if you have jowls or a double chin.

■ **If you have a high forehead,** apply a little soft brown powder or bronzing powder around the hairline to lessen the effect.

■ **Blusher doesn't have to be for your cheeks alone.** You can add a subtle glow to your whole face if you know where to put it. A dot on your chin, on the brow bones and even on your earlobes in summer (they often look a little pink during cold winter months) makes skin look radiant.

■ **Always use too little** rather than too much blusher.

■ **Build up the intensity of your blusher a little at a time.** When you're in a hurry, it's easy to apply too much, then try to rub off the excess afterwards. However, when you do rub off the excess colour, you bring the natural colour of your cheeks rushing to the surface, so you'll still look as though you've applied too much. And when your colour has gone down again, you'll find that you've removed all your blusher and look too pale!

lips

The size and shape of your mouth can have a profound effect on the way people see you. A full pouting mouth is perceived as more sexy, whereas someone with a thin or uneven mouth is often believed to be mean spirited.

changing the shape of your mouth

With a little expert help, lip colour can subtly change the shape of your mouth and create illusions, from a pert little Cupid's bow to a full, strong outline. When you're changing the natural shape of your mouth, don't try to alter the entire lip line – the fakery will just look more and more obvious as the colour fades away. You can block out your natural shape using a foundation stick or concealer to match the surrounding skin tone. Then practise with lip pencil, drawing in the shape you want, going inside or outside the natural line. However, never go too far. Minor adjustments done thoughtfully and carefully are far more convincing.

Corrections are also most effective if you use a subdued colour, such as matte medium tones, in your natural lip colour. Steer clear of red: it is one of the worst shades to use because it's so bright it draws attention to the mouth, and will show up a false lip shape.

if you have thin lips

Most of us would like to have a fuller mouth, especially as we get older and lips naturally get thinner. But try to avoid creating a lip line where you'd like it to be, rather than where it should be – you'll only end up looking like a clown. The best way to enhance lips is to apply a layer of light-reflective concealer (such as Yves Saint Laurent's famous Touche Eclat) all over the lip area and onto the skin. It will magically illuminate the whole area and make it appear bigger. Then draw your lip line with a firm pencil just a fraction beyond the natural edge of the lips, and soften the edge of the line so that it looks as soft and natural as possible. Finally, fill the whole area in with a medium matte shade of lipstick, and add a dab of gloss to the centre of the bottom lip to make it appear bigger, more rounded and full.

dental care

Even the most perfectly applied lip colour can't hide terrible teeth. Indeed, certain shades of lipstick (red, for example) can show up problems such as discoloration even more. Compared to our American cousins, for whom regular bleaching is almost the norm, we have a lot to learn. Make sure you brush regularly for a full two minutes, and visit a hygienist for regular cleaning. Take greater care of what you've got: prevention, in dentistry, is far better than cure.

Lip essentials

■ **'To prevent a harsh lip line,** always line your lips after applying lipstick,' says Daniel Sandler. 'This way the pencil will blend more easily, won't stand out and look obvious, and gives a softer finish to older mouths.'

■ **'I never use lip liner on thin lips,'** says Maggie Hunt. 'Instead, keep the shape undefined and glossy with a hint of light pastel colour to make them appear bigger.'

■ **'Apply lots of lip balm before you go to bed,'** says Laura Mercier. 'It works well while you are asleep, so in the morning your lips are really soft and supple.'

■ **Practise smiling more often.** It will brighten up and accentuate your looks. Try this exercise: keeping your mouth slightly open, smile repeatedly every second, 20 or 30 times. This will strengthen your jaw muscles and prevent the sides of your mouth from turning down.

■ **Lips lose their natural plumpness and colour** with age so outlining them gives extra definition. The ideal lip pencil needs to be firm enough to enable you to reshape an uneven outline, yet smooth enough to blend well on your lips. Most popular brands of lip liners with make-up artists include those by MAC, Nars and Shu Uemura.

■ **Don't think that chubby lip pencils create a good lip contour.** They are too wide and have a creamier formulation that will smudge. Leave them in your handbag for emergency colour only.

■ **'In warm climates,** submerge lip pencils (with caps on) in iced water to keep the tips firm,' says Laura Mercier.

■ **To check how well you've drawn your lip line,** wrap a cotton pad in a tissue and blot your lips with it. Then match up the outline to see just how precise your application has been.

make-up solutions

Here are the answers to some niggling beauty problems.

■ **If you find the price of lipsticks too hard to bear** and can't face throwing out the old lipstick stubs, do what the make-up artists do. Get a small tin or old eye-shadow compact and scoop out the remaining lip colour. Then simply apply with your fingertips for a soft, undefined mouth or with a lip brush for more precision.

■ **Caught without your lipstick?** Rub on a little rosy blusher, or some toffee-coloured eye-shadow then seal with lip balm.

■ **If your lipstick bleeds and feathers.** Vertical lines and wrinkles (the kind that appear with age) can siphon off even the most carefully applied lip colour. Your best bet is to prepare the skin around the mouth first with a moisturiser to smooth out the lines. Then use a lip pencil to define the outline of your lips and give the lipstick something else to cling to, and powder your lips well before and after applying lip colour. There are a number of lip bases and primers you can buy to help prevent feathering, but it's an extra step in a busy schedule, and many of these products can be drying to the lips.

■ **If you don't like your lips,** just use a gloss on them and accentuate the eyes more instead.

■ **If you suffer from high colour** but want to apply blusher, try calming redness or red veins with a hint of concealer, then choose a tawny peach blusher rather than a pink shade which has too much red in it. Remember, less is more: you're better off living with high colour than trying to hide it completely, or skin will just end up looking grey.

■ **If you've blobbed your mascara,** use a clean, damp mascara wand to separate clogged lashes and a damp cotton bud to clean blobs from the skin.

■ **If your mascara always smudges,** leave it off the bottom lashes. If it still smudges, it might not be a good formulation, so try buying a different make. Ask friends for their recommendations.

■ **If your eyes smart after using your regular eye make-up,** it's probably time to throw it out. Mascaras only tend to last around three months at the most.

■ **If you find that you are suddenly becoming sensitive around the eyes in general,** it may not necessarily be your eye make-up. A number of nail polishes contain irritants such as toluene and formaldehyde. If you are sensitive, you are more likely to develop a rash around the eyes where you've been touching them than around the nail.

■ **If you always get a wobbly line** when you apply eyeliner, keep your elbows steady on a table while looking down into a mirror, and stretch the skin along the lid before applying, so you have a smooth surface. Don't give up – practise makes perfect.

■ **To help low eyebrows appear higher,** brush eyebrows downwards so you can see exactly where the uppermost hairs emerge from the skin. With a pencil or eye-shadow and brush, trace along this upper limit, emphasising the highest part of your brow line, and when you brush the hairs up you'll neatly hide the pencilled line.

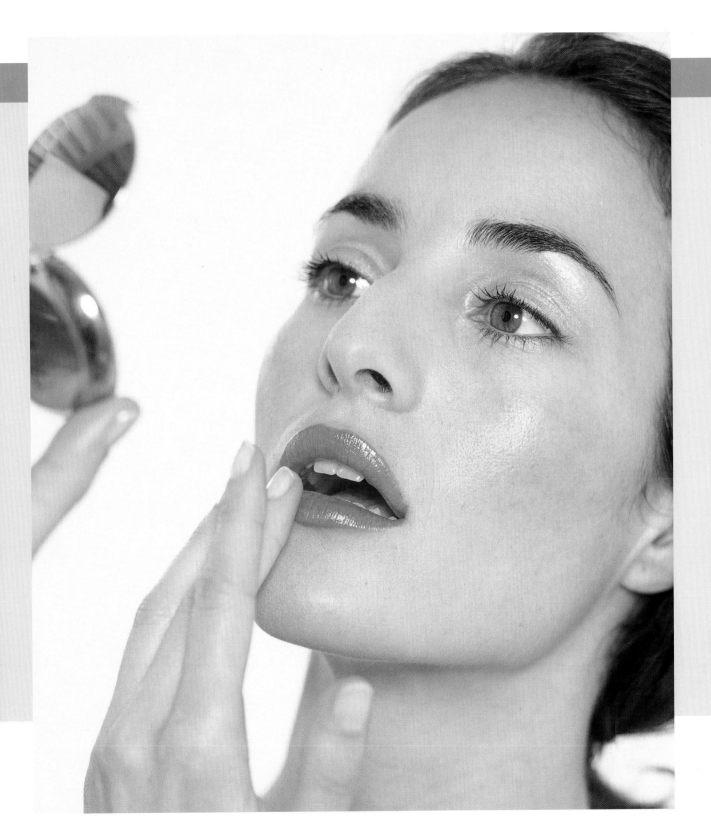

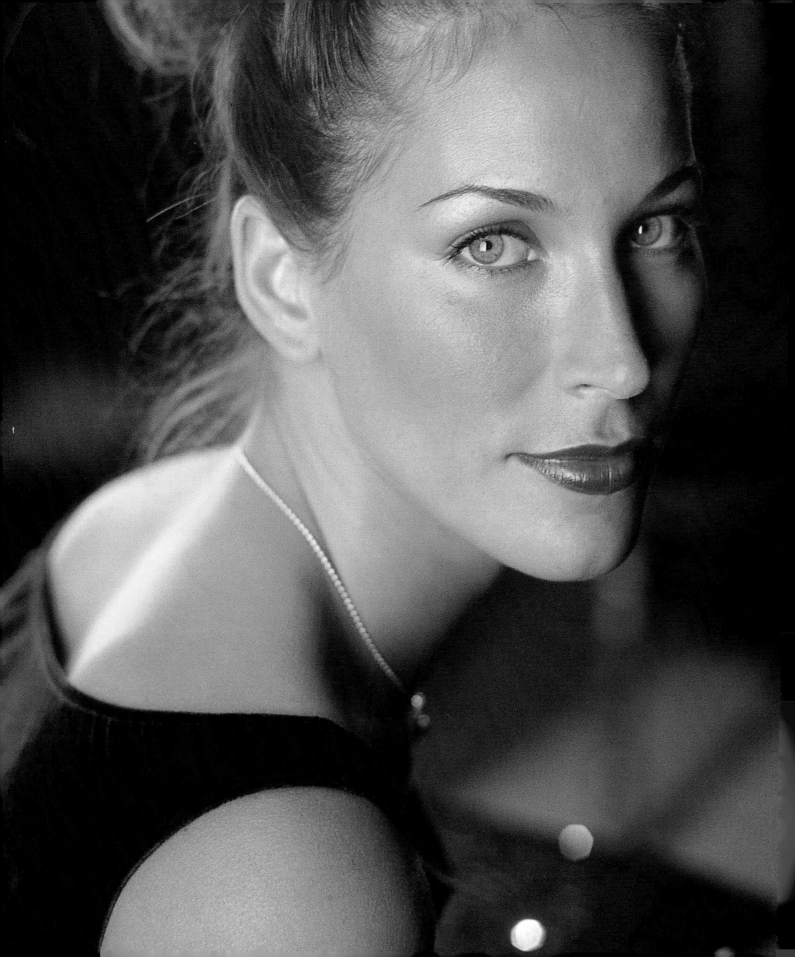

radiance make-up for nights

what's going on

It's hard enough to get your make-up looking great every single day of the week, but when you need a little more oomph for a special occasion, it's easy to overdo it and get it all wrong. Here are some key steps to getting it right.

foundation

The texture of your skin is the most important thing about your make-up,' says Cheryl Phelps-Gardiner. 'When your skin looks good, everything else looks good around it.' Make-up artists are totally obsessed with perfect skin – rare though it is. Watching Cheryl applying foundation is like watching an artist at work. She uses a fine brush dipped in a perfectly matched foundation, and literally paints out all imperfections. Skin looks its best when you only cover up what you need to, leaving the rest of your skin looking fresh. 'Try to leave your cheeks free from foundation for a more youthful look to your base. After applying foundation, wipe your cheeks so they keep as much natural colour showing as possible.'

eye concealer

Every woman over a certain age needs eye concealer. But not just any ordinary one. Cheryl's favourite is Yves Saint Laurent's light-reflective concealer *Touche Eclat* which lightens and brightens the 'dark' around the eyes rather than covering it up with a heavy layer of traditional cream concealer. 'You can ladle this on your skin and it still won't look as if you've overdone it,' she says. 'And unlike other concealers, *Touche Eclat* remains creamy for long enough so you can work it into place before it dries.' Apply eye concealer by looking straight ahead into a mirror and lowering your chin. Apply concealer to the dark areas only. Pat lightly to leave an even layer on the skin.

powder

If you need powder, use it just along the T-zone – the centre of the forehead, nose and chin– leaving the rest bare. 'These areas are where you want your skin to shine,' says Cheryl. If you suffer from skin redness or flushing, do try to live with it, rather than slavishly covering it up

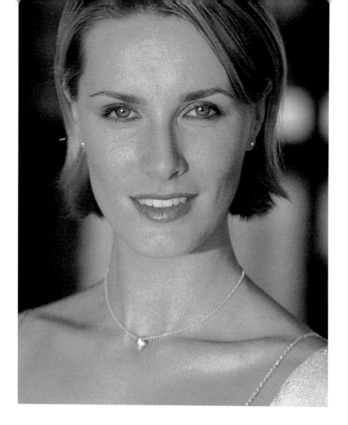

with coloured powders. These only make skin look grey and grimy. Try to tone redness in with a bronzing powder or a tawny coloured blusher instead. This way it looks like intended colour, rather than purely redness.

blusher

Cheryl prefers creamy blushers to powder ones. 'They are far more flattering on mature skin because they put the bloom back into skin, making it appear more dewy and fresh.' Start on the apple of your cheek, slowly working it outwards, diffusing it at the edges so it blends away. If you don't want to buy a new blusher, use a pinky rose lipstick in the same way.

shimmer

If you like shimmer on your cheeks, try mixing a little creamy highlighter in with your blusher on the back of your hand, or just pat a little shimmer along the tops of your cheekbones. Place it only on smooth areas of skin which don't have lines and wrinkles, to give a plump, rounded look. For a ready-made indispensable shimmer in a stick, nothing beats Nars' The Multiple. Stroke it over shoulders and the collarbone too.

eye-shadow

Prime eyes first with translucent powder to help eye-shadow last. Then, for the prettiest party eyes, apply a neutral powder eye-shadow all over the upper eyelids. Next, add a hint of pearlescent powder, using a fine, controllable brush (ie with short bristles), and place a little sparkle on the inner corners of the eyes where it brightens them up. Then place a fine vertical stripe down the centre of the upper eyelid to give the effect of shiny bright eyes, but without the risk of it going crepey during the evening and sinking into the creases.

eyeliner and mascara

Applied well, eyeliner gives evening make-up the edge. Liquid liner is quick and handy and gives a very definite line, but can look harsh. To soften it, Cheryl suggests drawing the line in powder first, lining over the top with a liquid liner or wet shadow/cake liner, then applying powder again over the top. If you'd rather stick to what you know best, the softest kohl pencils give the smudgiest, smokiest effect of all. Finish off with lashings of mascara. Wipe the wand with a tissue first to ensure lashes are separated. If you find your lashes are fine or sparse, Cheryl suggests filling in with a little black eye pencil inside the upper lashline to create the illusion of thicker, darker lashes.

eyebrows

Your eyebrows define your face and are a vital part of your make-up. You can make your evening make-up look more elegant simply by elongating your eyebrows. Fill in any blanks if they are sparse with a good firm, waxy crayon, follow the arch of your brow up, then carry the line out, finishing it just beyond where your brow naturally tapers off.

lips

You can afford to play up your lips a bit more. Moisturise them well first. Shape your lips with a natural toned lip pencil. Use to lightly define the natural shape of your lips, then diffuse with a clean cotton bud. Now apply colour – using a lip brush, straight from the tube, or with your finger. Make it a rich plum, which suits pretty much every woman, and finish off with a dab of gloss in the centre of both the top and bottom lips.

party tips

■ **Make the skin on your body as appealing as the skin on your face.** Models and actresses swear by Lancome's Maquisuperbe highlighting fluid as the key to sexy, sheeny skin. Cheryl recommends it for hands too. 'It's also great over hand cream, so that when you're talking in the candlelight and your hands are under your chin or by your face, they catch the light and look beautiful too.'

■ **If you are going to wear false eyelashes,** use individual ones. That way, if they fall out, it's just one that can be innocently brushed away, rather than a whole set.

■ **Brighten up your smile.** Whether with a piece of lemon rubbed across your teeth to remove the yellowness, or with a tooth-brightening toothpaste, it's one way to be more dazzling.

■ **A dot of shimmery silver shadow** on the inside corners of the eyes makes them sparkle and can instantly transform day make-up into glamour.

■ **Adding a light eye-shadow or shimmer eye pencil along the eyelids** instantly creates definition in the eye sockets without trying too hard.

Evening essentials

As evening bags become even smaller than your purse, there are a few evening essentials that are worth popping in alongside your door keys and credit card.

■ A tiny phial of your favourite perfume won't take up much space and acts as a great pick-me-up during an evening.

■ Keep a small bottle of eye drops (depending on whether or not you wear contact lenses) to refresh your eyes in smoky environments.

■ Little books of oil-blotting sheets are always good to have hand in your evening bag.

■ A tube of Lancôme T-Controle can be applied over your make-up base along the T-zone, so touch-ups to reduce shine are easy.

■ Carry a clear gloss to add sexy shine that catches the light at night and looks pretty on lips and cheeks, even with nothing else at all.

your hair

good day or bad day, your hair

is the one thing you just

can't hide. That's why it is so

vital to our self-esteem

and self-confidence. Its style

and colour has a profound

effect on our psyche

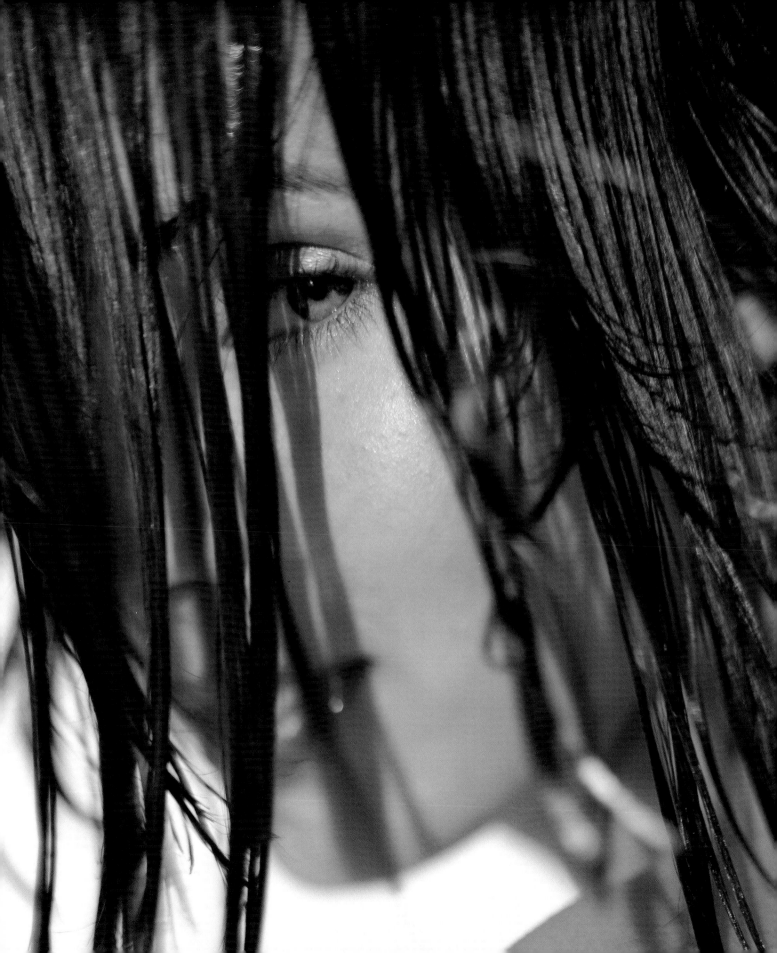

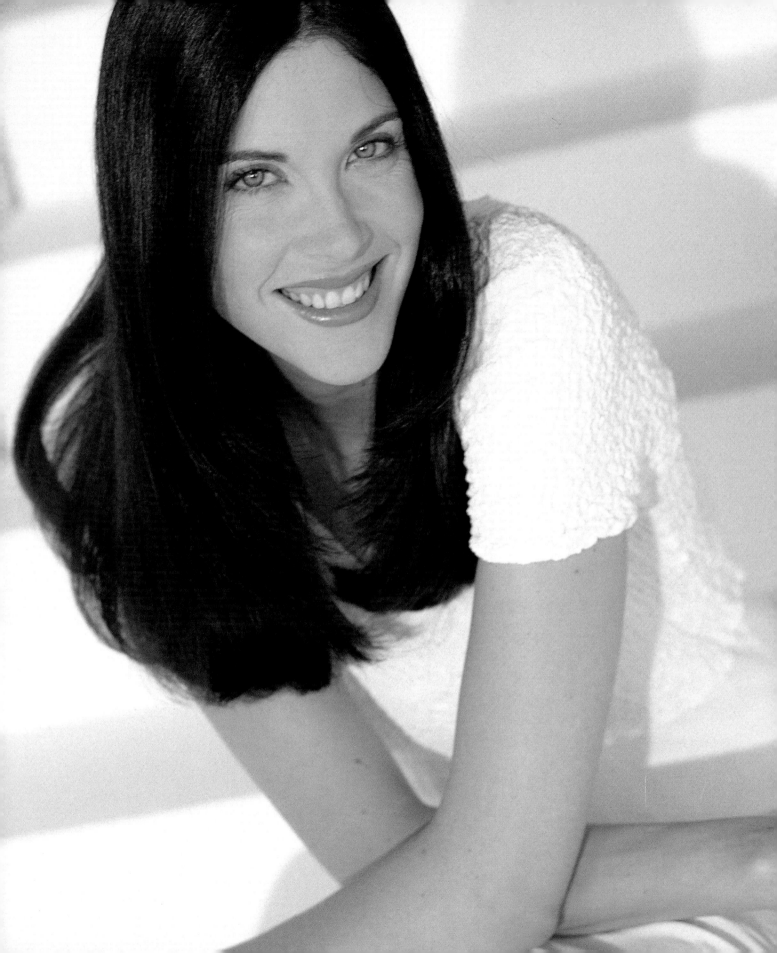

how and why
hair ages

what's going on

Just like your skin, your hair is affected by the way you live your life and the way you treat it. Years of abuse from the elements – sun, wind, water – and poor diet take their toll.

scalp problems

'Your hair is a true reflection of your health from within,' says Glen Lyons, consultant trichologist at Philip Kingsley Trichological Clinic in London. 'A great cut and all the styling products in the world can't mask damage caused by physical or psychological stress and poor nutrition; and your scalp is the first place to show the signs of distress. If the body needs to conserve vital nutrients to cope with illness, stress or bad diet, the first place it stops supplying is the scalp.' Not surprisingly, we take more notice of skin problems, which are on show, than scalp problems which are often hidden. And we'd be far more inclined to visit a doctor or dermatologist than a trichologist.

hair structure

Hair grows from the follicle, deep in the skin's lower layer, and is nourished by its own blood supply. Like skin, hair cells move upward from the roots as they mature (over 28 days) so that the visible part of the hair shaft is made up entirely of dead keratin scales, called cuticles, the same as the skin's surface layer (called the stratum corneum). All cell division slows down in the mid-thirties and at this time a number of hair follicles become inactive, By the time you reach your fifties, the number may well have halved.

We're all born with a genetically predetermined number of follicles (around 120,000) and the size of the follicle determines the hair's thickness. Hair grows half an inch a month, on average, though faster in summer than winter. The rate of hair growth is controlled by the body's hormones, and there are always new hairs on the way to replace hair that is naturally shedding – normally up to 100 hairs a day.

In women, oestrogen prevents hair from growing on the face and diverts it to the head. We may benefit from this at a younger age, especially during pregnancy, with generally thicker, more lustrous hair than men, However, after giving birth, and when oestrogen levels drop during the menopause, hair becomes noticeably thinner and many women may begin to experience hair loss.

hair health

Your hair can so easily reflect how you feel from the way it looks. When it looks great, you feel fantastic but when it looks bad, you feel even worse because it's all on show and there's little you can do to hide it.

why hair shines

Healthy hair is shiny hair. It shines because the protective coating of each hair shaft, the cuticle, lies flat, creating a smooth surface to reflect the light brilliantly. The flatter and tighter the cuticles, the smoother the surface of the hair. And the smoother the hair, the shinier it will be. That's the ideal, but when the cuticles are repeatedly roughened and damaged through everyday treatment (over-processing, over-heating and poor conditioning) or are covered by a film of dirt, dust, soap residue or styling products, these cuticles become raised, peel and break, light is no longer reflected evenly, and hair becomes fragile and just looks dull.

The good news is that hair health is pretty much in our own hands. Care for your hair as you do your skin: cleanse it gently, moisturise (condition) it when needed, protect it from the sun (especially if hair is coloured or processed) and give it regular once-a-week pampering treats to keep it looking its best.

to boost shine

■ **Keep it clean** Clean hair is shiny. While, in theory, oil looks shiny, oily hair attracts dirt and dust from around us like a magnet, robbing hair of its shine. Wash it frequently (city hair needs washing more often due to pollution and dust): no more than two or three days between shampoos, especially if you use a variety of styling products.

■ **Change your shampoo** Use a mild shampoo regularly, then every couple of weeks try a residue cleansing shampoo to refresh the hair and remove product build-up.

■ **Moisturise it** Damaged cuticles are rough. Moisturising conditioners, shampoos and styling products can attract and bind moisture to the hair, smoothing the cuticle and boosting shine at the same time. Remember, water and oil are two separate things: your hair needs both.

■ **Condition** It not only smoothes and seals the outer cuticle, but protects hair from further damage from sun and styling products until the next time you wash. Warm up half a teacup of olive oil, comb through, avoiding the scalp, and leave on for five minutes, then shampoo out and condition as normal. All hair types need conditioner.

■ **Straighten it** Curly hair is less shiny than straight hair because straight reflects the light while curls absorb it. Set wavy and curly hair on heated rollers to boost shine.

■ **Control the frizz** When hair frizzes, light is scattered rather than uniformly reflected. Try a post-shampoo conditioner, a leave-in conditioner or a frizz tamer.

■ **Use the right brush** Natural bristles are best for smoothing and grabbing the hair, aligning individual strands and promoting more shine.

■ **Slow down** Drying too fast blows individual hairs around unnecessarily, so the cuticles are more likely to get ruffled and therefore reduce shine.

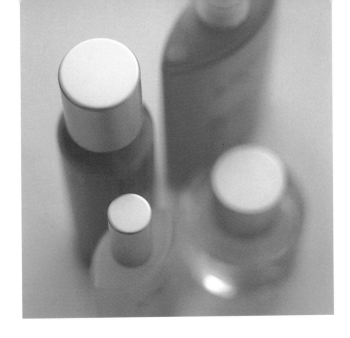

■ **Make waves** Setting hair on big rollers realigns individual strands so they lie together, making a larger, smoother surface for reflecting light.

■ **Use silicone** Serums are silicone-based products that add shine no matter what your hair type. Apply to towel-dried hair and add a little bit more after styling, once dry, for extra shine. But don't go overboard. If you use more than a couple of drops, hair will instantly become limp, heavy and greasy looking.

■ **Protect it** Hair is exposed on a daily basis to the environment: sun, wind, rain, sea, pollution, chlorinated water – chemicals that roughen the surface texture and reduce shine and lustre. At the very least, wear a hat in extremes of weather and when swimming.

■ **Cut cleverly** Layers absorb shine. The fewer layers you have in your hair, the shinier it will look.

scalp matters

There are three classic types of scalp problems: a dry scalp, oily scalp and dandruff, which can exist with both but is far more common in an oily scalp. A dry scalp can be due to your genes, or a change in weather. An oily scalp can be caused by too much oil being created in the sebaceous glands or inadequate cleansing. Dandruff is referred to as a 'non-inflammatory scaliness of the scalp' and is often the result of stress, poor circulation and bad diet – common to most of us between the age of 19 and

45. Stress is a big factor in scalp problems. Conditions get significantly better on holiday: hair is shampooed more frequently, diet improves (more fresh fruits and salads), and UV exposure is therapeutic.

Scalp problems are closely linked to skin problems – the scalp being skin. If you find that you have a problem scalp, you should seek advice from a trichologist (hair doctor) or a dermatologist. Pityriasis amiantacea (PA) is a scaling on the scalp, much like cradle cap in babies and young children, only thicker, and is due to excessive oiliness. According to Glen Lyons, consultant at the Philip Kingsley Trichological Clinic, it is the only scaly scalp condition that causes hair loss. Stress is a common factor in scalp problems. Acupuncture and reflexology are both very effective relaxation techniques for stress-related itchy, sensitive scalps.

to improve the condition of your scalp

■ **Frequent washing:** wash every day or every other day with a mild shampoo. Avoid medicated shampoos which are often too strong and tar-based shampoos which can be too dry.

■ **Improve your diet:** cut down on white wine and dairy products, which can aggravate sensitive skin conditions such as eczema, psoriasis and dandruff.

■ **Relax:** acupuncture is very effective for stress-related itchy, sensitive scalps.

■ **True inflammatory scaling of the scalp** is psoriasis and affects less than 3 per cent of the population. Here, instead of the skin cells on the scalp turning over every 28 days, as on the face, it's every 48 hours. In this case the only way to control it is UV exposure and 'manual shifting'. This is often carried out by a doctor or trichologist, and is achieved by massaging a little oil into the scalp then gently brushing off the flakes with a small, soft brush.

can you really turn back the clock?

Looking after your hair is one of the best ways to turn back the clock. By boosting its colour, condition and cut, and finding the right style to suit you, you will undoubtedly find new confidence and self-esteem.

hair length

Is long hair, past a certain age, ageing? When you get older, long hair can create a curtain that hangs around the face, pulling the features (and slackening facial contours) downwards, which invariably makes it appear to be more ageing. However, that doesn't mean you shouldn't – and can't – get away with having long hair as you get older. 'Condition is the most crucial thing,' says Neil Cornelius of stylists Michaeljohn. 'Think of Goldie Hawn. If your hair is looked after properly, you can still get away with wearing it long whatever your age.' Clever layers can help you to create a mid-length feel, while still keeping the overall length. It can also boost essential body and help make long hair surprisingly easier to style.

'Short hair is often harder work than you'd imagine, though women often perceive it as the first choice beyond a "certain age". Each morning it either lies flat, or sticks out in all directions; needs cutting every four weeks, not six or eight the way you'd prefer; and it's hard to colour yourself at home.'

Medium hair is neither short nor long, and however you style it, it inevitably still manages to look like a bob. But it's the ideal length whatever your age, because it combines the convenience of short hair with the glamour of long hair. And any hair texture works well at this length, because it's still easy enough to make sleek and straight or add volume and curls. Just vary the style by layering the ends and chopping into it a bit, and you'll get more of a low-maintenance, relaxed and casual chic look that's fashionable and very wearable.

going grey

Going grey is inevitable, but some of us are genetically predisposed to go grey much earlier than others, even in late teens and early 20s. Hair gets its colour from pigment produced by the cells (called melanocytes) in the hair follicles. With age these cells become less active and colour fades and appears grey. Hair eventually turns white when these cells cease altogether. A diet lacking in the essential hair vitamin B, depleted by stress, has also been found to accelerate grey. If in doubt, seek professional advice and bump up your intake of vitamin B. Whether you are a readhead, blonde or brunette – or somewhere in between – hair colour can often reveal a great deal about your personality and, when hair turns grey, we often feel as if we've lost our identity. That is one reason why it is important to be comfortable with your hair colour. If you aren't happy, you should seek advice from your hairdresser about colourants.

hair loss

Hair loss is common among women, but it is rarely talked about. According to trichologist Glen Lyons, stress is a major factor in hair loss as it triggers the male

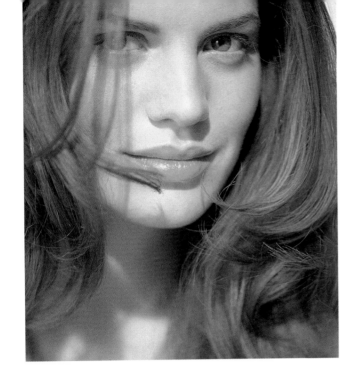

hormone testosterone, which is the main cause of baldness in men. In addition, the very factors that cause our hair to look tired, dull and lacking in lustre – poor diet, illness, prescription drugs, physical and chemical over-processing, and lack of protection from the elements – eventually weaken the follicles.

anti-ageing haircare

Look for all the latest skincare ingredients in your hair-care, too. Antioxidant vitamins C and E will help to protect against oxidisation which fades hair colour fast. UVA and UVB sun filters prevent dehydration, splitting and breakage from UV exposure. Enzymes and AHAs in shampoos help to cleanse hair deep down to remove product build-up and leave hair shiny; proteins (such as keratin, the hair protein) and amino-acid complexes help to smooth, strengthen and rebuild the hair cuticle.

essential daily haircare

'Nine out of ten hair problems are self-inflicted,' says Glen Lyons. 'Vibrant, glossy, younger-looking hair shines because its cuticles lie smooth and reflect the light perfectly.' But when repeatedly damaged by heat, chemicals or just some rough handling, these cuticles become raised, peel and break, so hair ultimately becomes more fragile and dull.

things to avoid

■ **using the hottest setting on your hairdryer.** This can burn the hair, making it dull, coarse and split. Leave it to dry naturally as often as you can, saving serious styling for hot dates only.

■ **brushing hair when it's wet** or it will pull, snag and split because it's too harsh and stretches hair beyond its elasticity. Only ever comb hair through when it's wet.

■ **leaving it too long between washes.** This makes hair dull because it's covered by a film of dust and dirt and styling products. Clean hair is shiny hair, so wash it more often. 'Don't leave it any longer than two or three days,' says Trevor Sorbie, 'especially if you use lots of styling products.'

'sexy hair is well-groomed but shouldn't look as if you've just stepped out of the hairdresser's. There's nothing seductive about someone who has tried too hard.'

Leading hairdresser Nicky Clarke

haircare tips

Insider tips from leading hairdressers that will make your hair look great.

■ **If your hair looks dull.** Change your shampoo. It refreshes your hair every time you swap, simply because it cleans differently, removing a different level of product build-up. Use a detox shampoo every three to four weeks to remove all build-up in your hair.

■ **'Just because your hair is long** it doesn't mean you can leave it without a trim for much longer than short hair. It keeps the sharpness about a cut, and reduces split ends.' Denise McAdam.

■ **Always start drying hair at the roots,** especially underneath at the nape of the neck because the hair here supports the style.

■ **When straightening,** use a leave-in conditioner and always use a medium heat setting. Think about it: once you iron a shine on a suit, you never lose it, and once you burn hair you won't lose it until you cut it out. And that's a long time if you have long hair.

■ **'If you like the effect of blow-drying** but can't bear to do it yourself, try using a hot airbrush instead. It dries hair thoroughly as you brush through, making it a lot easier to manage single-handedly than a hairdryer. Remember, only start styling with hair that is already 80 per cent rough dried, otherwise you'll take forever and end up using a lot more heat, which causes more damage.' Nicky Clarke.

■ **'Remember, when curling** – whether on ordinary rollers or bendi-rollers, that create a tighter curl – the larger the section of hair wrapped round, the bigger the curl. And always tuck the ends neatly under to ensure smooth ends.' Charles Worthington.

■ **A couple of well-placed rollers** on the crown can help boost volume at the roots, even when hair is very straight and flat. Choose 'flocked' heated rollers which are covered in velvet, making them gentler because they don't grab at hairs. Blow-dry all over to increase the drying speed, and always allow the rollers to cool right down before you remove them. Then spray over to keep in the root lift.

■ **'For an instant style reviver,** tip your head upside down, spray the roots with a styling spray, allow to dry, then throw back your head.' Nicky Clarke.

■ **'If your highlights repeatedly tend to look yellow,** brassy and dull after just a few weeks, it may be caused by the metals in the water you wash it in. Always protect colour in the sun: it lightens and dehydrates hair, fading colour fast, and puts extra wear and tear on your hair. Save having your highlights done until after you come back, letting the sun's natural lightening take effect, so you need less colour added. And brighten up highlights with detox shampoos and brightening products.' Sally Hershenberger at John Frieda.

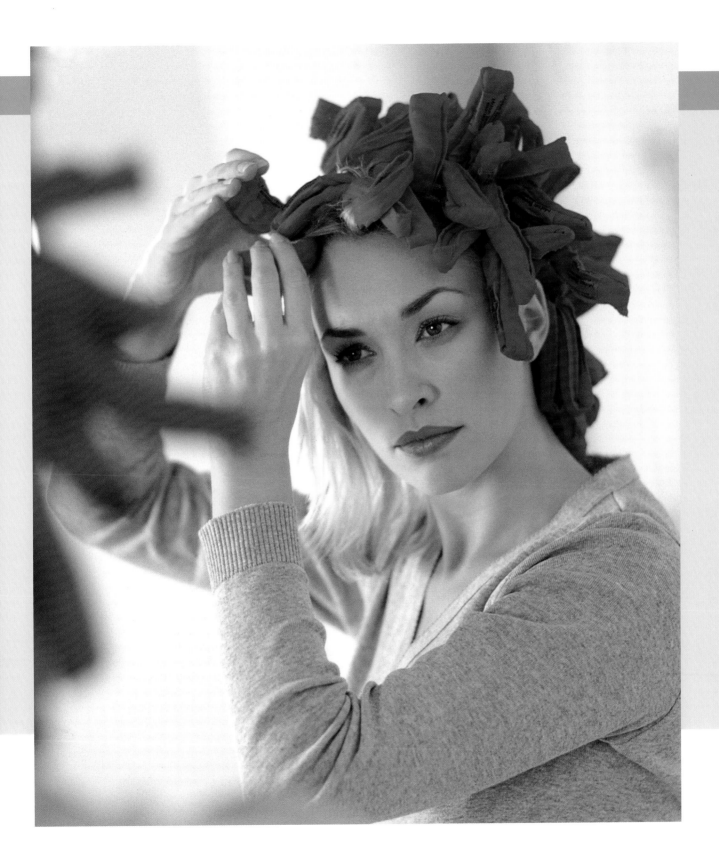

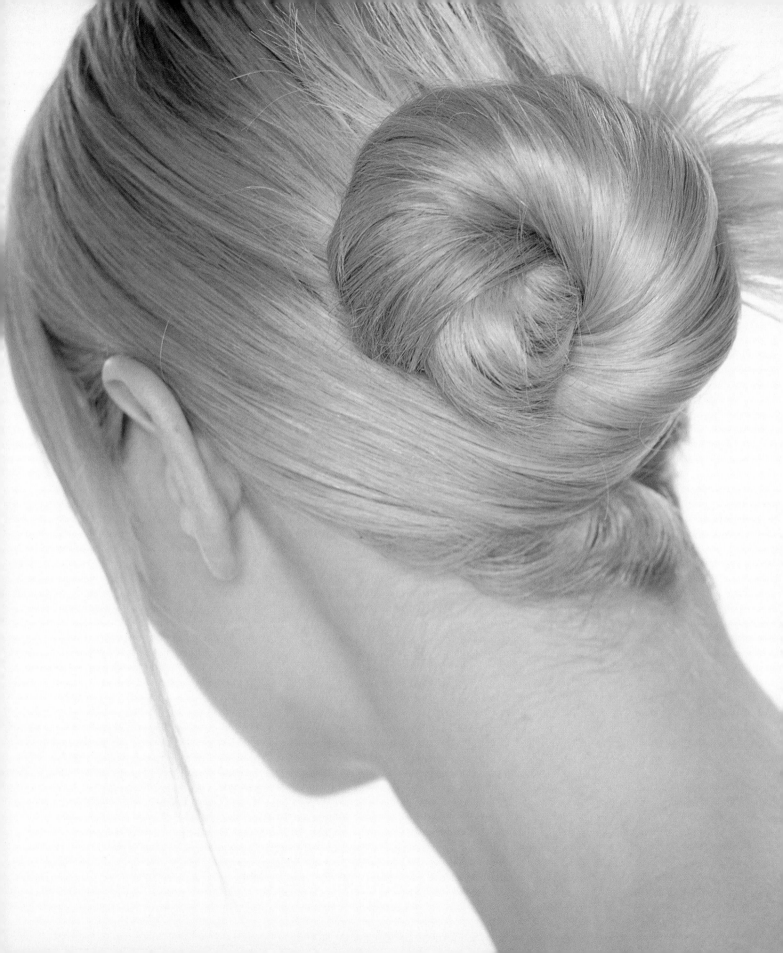

daily hair
requirements

why great hair matters

On a bad hair day we're not happy with our hair or ourselves. On a good day, we're much more confident. Find a hairstyle that works for your hair and put an end to bad hair days.

stop fighting it

Too curly, too straight. Too thick, too thin. Rarely are any of us happy with our own hair. But guess what – no matter what type of hair you've got, there's always someone with the opposite who's willing to swap! So now's the time to stop fighting it, straightening it, perming. Learn to live with your hair, rather than trying to change it. Experts believe that the hair texture you're born with is the one that suits you best. So find a style that works with your hair the way it really is, then see variations as a perk.

accentuate the positive

Leading hairdresser Charles Worthington says: 'Women with fine hair usually think a perm is the only answer, because all they see is that their hair is too flat. What they really need is a good cut. Fine hair shines like no other, especially if you give it a smooth cut. Those with very curly hair often want to relax it to achieve a more groomed, polished look. But it's worth remembering that natural curls have more body and life than anything you'd ever get from a perm. Separate and smooth the curls with a little serum, then leave the hair to air dry.'

go with what you've got

Women with very dense hair sometimes ask to have it thinned. Instead, blow dry with a little setting lotion, and appreciate the fact that you have the fullness and body that everyone else is desperate to achieve. When women are dissatisfied with their hair, they often consider a drastic colour change. It is often better to get a cut that will make the most of your natural hair colour, so the upkeep is less demanding. For example, a blunt cut will play up the shine of dark hair, while soft layers will add movement and show off natural highlights in summer.

People with coarse, wiry hair don't realise that fullness can work to their advantage when they get a beautiful layered cut that won't go flat, whereas women with baby fine hair don't appreciate the fact that their hair is swingy, healthy and shiny. Save yourself time and money by making the most of what you've got.

shampoo and conditioner

Clean hair is shiny hair. Wash it frequently, especially if you live or work in the city. And use conditioner, which is basically a moisturiser for your hair. As with face creams, the older you get, the more necessary this becomes.

how often to shampoo

Frequently if your hair is fine, thin, oily or you suffer from scalp problems. The tendency is to leave well alone for as long as possible when there's a problem, but provided you use a mild, frequent use shampoo, you should be able to wash it daily. Dilute your shampoo with water before applying it to your hair. If, however, your hair is dry (and your scalp isn't especially oily) over-shampooing can remove essential natural oils so you can afford to leave it for two to three days.

how to choose

Follow this golden rule: choose a shampoo for your scalp and conditioner for your hair, especially if your scalp tends to be either excessively dry or oily. The idea is that while you need to clean the scalp, the hair shaft doesn't really get very dirty. But hair ends get no oils to speak of, so the hair itself, rather than your scalp, should dictate which conditioner you need.

how to shampoo

If you have a normal scalp, concentrate on your scalp for the first application of shampoo, then with the second, massage the suds into your hair. If you have a dandruff-prone scalp, make sure you rinse off every speck of shampoo. Use clear, running water and don't skimp. Insufficient rinsing is a common reason for dull hair. Wash combs and brushes as often as you wash your hair.

shampoo tips

■ **Thoroughly wet hair** needs less shampoo to get it clean, so don't skimp on water.

■ **It's a myth that shampoo should foam** – but it's a hard one to get over if you like the effect of lathering up all those bubbles. If your hair is squeaky clean, chances are that it is not just clean but probably dried out.

■ **Rinse through with vinegar.** A final 'vinegar rinse' (one part vinegar to 20 parts water) removes shampoo and styling product residue, both of which can make hair appear dull. The acidity of the vinegar also tightens the cuticles of the hair, making it look shinier.

■ **Vary your shampoo.** You know from experience that it refreshes your hair every time you swap. Then every three weeks use a detox shampoo to remove build-up from styling products. You may need to change your shampoo seasonally too, as the scalp can get more oily during warm summer months.

■ **If you feel the need to wash your hair every day, do so.** Washing doesn't make hair fall out and won't make it any drier.

■ **You don't need to shampoo twice with every wash.** Only do this if you have a build-up of styling products or residue in your hair that requires extra cleansing.

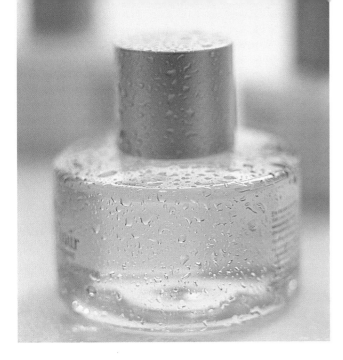

how often to condition

Conditioning your hair every time you shampoo not only smoothes and seals the outer cuticle, but provides daily protection from environmental damage. All hair needs conditioner – just apply to the tips and keep away from the scalp if your hair is oily or fine.

how to choose

Choose your conditioner for the state of your hair, whether it is dry, dull or normal. For dry, unmanageable hair, after applying conditioner blot your hair with a towel but don't rub it. Lank, dull hair also needs conditioning to give it body. Massage conditioner into the tips. A leave-in conditioner is ideal for those with dry hair, afro hair, or dry ends. An intensive conditioner acts like a monthly mask, and not only smoothes and seals the cuticle shut, but also protects your hair from further damage, whether it's from the sun or your hairdryer.

how to condition

Although it may depend on the type of conditioner you choose, experts recommend leaving a rinse-off conditioner on your hair for at least two minutes – longer if your hair is very dry. The most important thing to ensure is that every strand of hair is coated evenly. Applying a little conditioner to the ends of very long hair before you shampoo will also help to keep it from tangling while you wash.

conditioning tips

■ **Always use conditioner on the ends of your hair** if it is medium to long in length. Gently comb through, and never brush hair through while it is wet.

■ **Once a month, use an intensive conditioning treatment** on your hair to help replace some of the moisture lost through blow-drying. It will leave your hair unbelievably soft and much more manageable.

■ **If your hair is fine,** lacks body and invariably goes flat after washing, avoid using a 2-in-1 shampoo and conditioner, as the residue of conditioner left behind will weight hair down even more. But don't avoid conditioner altogether. Wash hair every day with a mild frequent wash shampoo, to keep the scalp clean and reduce oiliness. Then use a separate lightweight conditioner on the ends.

■ **Make your own rich conditioner** to treat a flaky scalp or dry hair. Mash half a ripe avocado and two drops of rosemary essential oil together with two tablespoons of olive oil, and blend together until it makes a smooth paste. Massage the mixture into your hair, wrap a warm towel around your head and leave on for 40 minutes to one hour. Shampoo thoroughly.

■ **Make sure you always thoroughly rinse conditioner out your hair** (unless, of course, it is designed to be left in). Excess residue on the hair shaft dulls the cuticles and makes hair look dull and dirty faster.

hairstyling essentials

The best styling equipment and products, whatever your hair type.

■ **Blow-dry styling cream** An indispensable styling product that is generally used prior to blow-drying, and in between washes as needed, to calm down 'fluffiness' in hair after blow-drying. It's a cream that looks and feels like a leave-in conditioner, and helps to replenish lost moisture from using the hairdryer, making it the perfect styling product for normal to dry hair.

■ **Comb** Vital to disperse conditioner evenly through the hair, and gently helps to detangle without stretching and snapping the hair. Choose a 'saw-cut' comb which is made from one piece of wood, metal or plastic and so has no rough edges which otherwise catch and snag hairs.

■ **Hairdryer** An easy to handle, lightweight hairdryer with a cool air setting, a covered vent and the right wattage for your hair type. Use a 1500 watt dryer for fine hair, 1600-1800 for thick hair.

■ **Hairspray** is a fine finishing spray that keeps hair in place after styling. All styles benefit from using a little hairspray, but limit its use if you have dry hair as its alcohol content can be drying.

■ **Hot air brush** This is ideal if you like the effect of blow-drying but can't bear to do it yourself. A good hot brush has a round head and dries hair smoothly as you brush through, making it a lot easier to manage single-handedly than a hairdryer. Most have interchangeable brushes and a nozzle, and flexible wide teeth to give better control over your hair.

■ **Mousse** gives body and shape to most hairstyles, and especially suits fine hair that needs volume without making the hair sticky.

■ **Pomade** gives soft styling and texture to layered hair without stickiness and is the modern alternative to wax, which can be heavy on the hair making it difficult to apply. Great for short, thick hair (curly or straight), unruly grey hair, and men's styles, it smoothes and slicks, adding definition and shine.

■ **Round brush,** often called a radial brush, with medium-length natural bristles which grip hair well, can be used to smooth, straighten and wave hair. The larger the head, the straighter it will make your hair; the smaller the head, the tighter the curl.

■ **Serum** is mainly silicone-based and forms a fine film on each hair shaft to help smooth and seal dry ends, calm frizziness and combat static. It leaves hair phenomenally shiny and healthy looking.

■ **Straightening irons** have flat metal plates which press together like an iron to flatten hair and smooth out unwanted kinks and curls. Great for certain styles which suit poker straight hair, but limit their use and keep them moving to minimise heat damage.

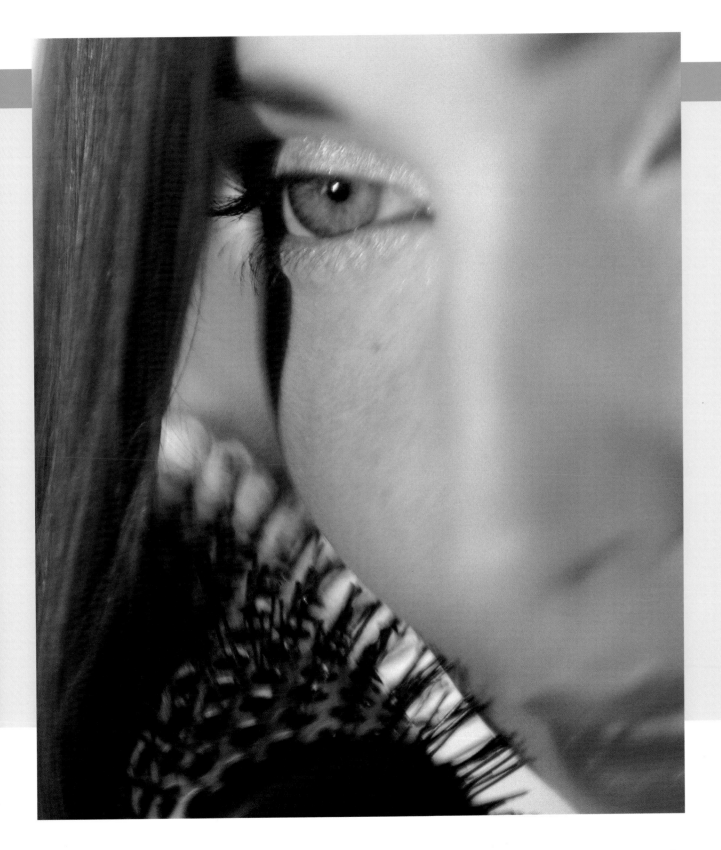

specialist haircare

Products that you can use at home to give your hair a professional finish.

■ **Mousse** Builds volume into the hair – something from which all hair types benefit, especially after a certain age. However, this lightweight styling product is best suited to those with fine hair: it gives extra body and hold without weighing hair down or making it sticky. For root lift, apply a ball of mousse between the palms, rub together and massage into the roots before blow-drying. To add body, apply to the mid section and the ends of your hair, comb through and blow dry.

■ **Styling spray** The modern equivalent of setting lotion, this forms a fine film on the hair which sets the style as it dries quickly. Many still contain alcohol which, although drying to hair, enables it to style fast. Suitable for any hair type that needs volume and root lift, especially fine or thinning hair.

Choose the right formulation for your particular hair type (normal, dry or oily). Once hair is almost dry, part it into small sections and apply directly to the roots, then finish off setting the style. Avoid using too much: setting lotions and sprays attract dirt very easily so hair will look dull, and it's easy to overdo it and end up with limp hair rather than body.

■ **Hair mask** Much like a face mask, this is simply a deep conditioning treatment for your hair that you leave on for between five and 20 minutes to bring condition and lustre back to hair. You can get deep cleansing masks which contain mud to help remove any residue of hair styling products; moisturising masks which help to replenish moisture and suppleness on dry ends; and protein masks which help to strengthen and 'rebuild' hair by conditioning the hair cuticle.

Once a month, apply to freshly washed hair which has had any excess water blotted out. Wrap a warm towel around your head and leave for the recommended amount of time. The additional warmth will ensure that your hair absorbs as much of the product as possible, making it that much more effective. Rinse thoroughly and style.

■ **Serum** comes in liquid or spray formulas and most are silicone based to add incredible shine and gloss, no matter what your hair type. It's best for normal to dry hair that's quite thick and feels a bit parched, especially on the ends. Those with oily or thin hair are better off with a volume product as silicone can easily weigh hair down, making matters worse.

Apply to towel-dried hair and add a little bit more after styling (once the hair is dry) for extra shine. But don't go overboard. If you use more than a couple of drops of serum, hair will instantly become limp, heavy and greasy looking. Apply a tiny amount after conditioner: too much will weigh your hair down.

your hair

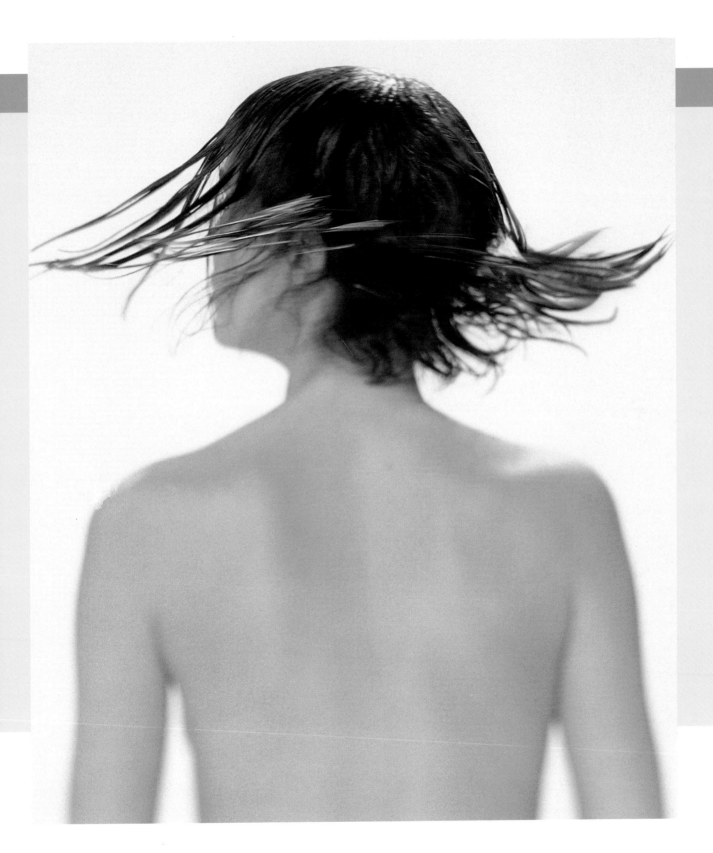

DIY hair salon

The upkeep of your hair in the salon doesn't come cheap. That's not to say don't go to the hairdresser, but there are a few tricks you might want to master at home to keep your hair looking good in between visits

the perfect blow-dry

Invariably we spend ages doing it, then don't end up drying it enough, either for fear of overdoing it or simply because we can't keep our arm in the air for that long! The result is that the shape doesn't last, and any unwanted frizziness and kinks that you've tried to smooth out come back.

how to do it

Rough dry your hair all over, until it's about 80 per cent dry. Never blow-dry hair from soaking wet: not only will it take too long (more heat means more damage), it over-stretches the hairs until they snap. Apply a small ball of mousse to help control any flyaway tendency, or a heat styling cream which calms down that fluffy blow-dried look. Always start drying the underneath layers first, around the nape of the neck. It supports the style, and prevents the top layers from drying out.

If you are blow-drying smooth and as straight as possible, use a large round radial brush with natural bristles which catch and hold hair better so you get more control.

Clip hair into sections no wider than the width of your brush. Don't move on to the next section until the one you're working on is totally dry. It's often easier to hold a hairdryer by the nozzle than by the handle.

Aim the dryer down the hair shaft, from roots to ends, to close and smooth the cuticle. Rub a tiny amount of shine product onto your fingertips to weigh hair down and reduce fluffiness, then smooth the rest over the surface.

cut your own fringe

Not for those with poor eyesight or an unsteady hand! This often seems such an easy thing to do yourself, but can so easily go wrong. And cutting your fringe without cutting the rest, unless it's long and all one length, can throw your style completely out of balance.

how to do it

Stylist Denise McAdam explains: 'If you must trim your own fringe between cuts, do it like this: get a small rubber band and secure the hair, with the band positioned between the eyes. Then "chip" into the ends, creating a "paintbrush" end. Always cut longer than you want, erring on the side of caution. This method cuts the fringe into a kind of half moon shape, gently curving at the edges, rather than going straight across and looking too severe and uneven.'

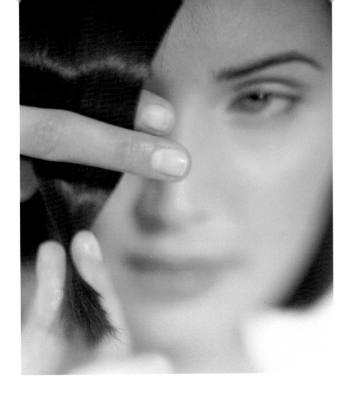

have a deep conditioning treatment

Perfect if your hair is dry from over-processing or too much sun, deep conditioning hair masks contain protein to help strengthen, moisturise and rebuild hair as the proteins become absorbed under the cuticles and fill any gaps.

how to do it

For best results, apply before going in the bath as the heat will open up the cuticles and allow the ingredients to become better absorbed. Apply to freshly washed, towel-dried hair which has had as much excess water blotted out as possible. Leave on hair for the recommended amount of time, depending on which product you choose (usually anything between 5–20 minutes) and wrap a sheet of clingfilm around your hair, then wrap up in a warm towel. Any additional warmth will ensure that your hair absorbs as much of the product as possible. Rinse thoroughly and if possible allow your hair to dry naturally without using a hairdryer.

create curls

Otherwise known as 'great body', those born with curly or wavy hair are often so busy trying to smooth, relax or straighten natural curls in order to get a more 'sophisticated and groomed' look that they can forget how versatile curly hair really is. So if they're natural, here's how to make the most of them.

how to do it

To enhance natural curls, adding a diffuser attachment to your hairdryer is the gentlest way. Choose a medium heat setting – high speed helps keep shine and reduce dryness but, if it's too hot, hair will be fluffy and dehydrated. For softer, smoother, tumbling waves, use heated rollers (the bigger the roller, the looser the curl). Lightly spray dry hair with spray gel or setting lotion first, comb through, then wind small sections of hair around each roller. Leave to cool, then remove each one. Avoid brushing your hair: simply apply a touch of serum to your fingers, then coax the end of each curl around your fingers to add gloss and definition.

For tighter, more defined curls, try flexible heated stylers. Spray hair with a little styling gel first, then wind a section of hair around the centre of the styler and bend it in the middle to secure it in place. Leave to cool, then remove and run fingers through to soften the curl.

If you want more permanent curls, don't try perming at home. Go to a reputable salon and take photos of the kind of curl you like so that the stylist stands a chance of getting it right. Only perm your hair if you really think you have no other choice. It rarely looks natural and, once the perm starts to grow out, it looks very obvious along the roots.

applying your own colour

Whether you want to cover up lots of grey, subtly perk up your natural colour or make a big sensation, nothing beats colour. The trick is to know what effect you want, know your limitations and be realistic about the results you can get from home – for example, if you have brown hair you won't go blonde with a 'wash in, wash out' colour tint.

how to do it

Unless you're going for a complete colour change, in which case you should see a professional hairdresser, keep within your own colour range for a more natural effect. If in doubt, choose the next shade lighter or deeper than your own. Make sure to put on protective gloves before you start.

For the best, even coverage: work colour in well from back to front, separating hair into two-inch sections as you go, rather than squeezing all over and then trying to spread it. If your hair is longer than chin length, don't apply colour directly onto the ends – they're drier and more porous, and will absorb more colour than you'll want. Leave on for the desired amount of time, then rinse thoroughly until water runs clear.

choose the right colourant

If you want to subtly alter your colour, choose colour that washes out quickly and works within the limits of your hair's natural shade.

■ **Temporary** – lasts for a couple of washes. These don't lighten or penetrate the hair, and often disappear the next time you shampoo. They are best for brightening your own natural colour, or for making a quick but temporary change that also helps to give you an idea of what shade to go for permanently.

■ **Semi-permanent** – lasts up to 8 washes. These coat the hair with colour but won't lighten it, so they will tint your natural shade, add some texture and body, and some condition too. They will also cover some grey, but not evenly, turning the grey strands into highlights instead.

If you want to dramatically alter your colour by three shades or more, then you need colour that is more permanent. These products work by lightening your natural hair colour first, before depositing a new colour on top. If you buy a colourant that involves mixing two solutions together, then rest assured it's going to last a while.

■ **Tone-on-tone** – lasts up to 24 washes. These work like semi-permanents except that most contain a low level of hydrogen peroxide to lighten hair, making the colour last three times longer. They work on any hair colour and fade gradually with each wash, reducing the undesirable 'roots' effect.

■ **Permanent** – lasts until it gets cut out. For dramatic, long-lasting colour changes and covering up a lot of grey, these work by lifting colour out of the hair and depositing a new shade instead. They work on any hair colour, but roots show through as soon as the colour starts to grows out. (Highlights are permanent colour, but tend to grow out more subtly because they only cover random strands of hair.) Repeated long term permanent colour is harder on the hair than any other type of colour and is not generally recommended for relaxed or permed hair.

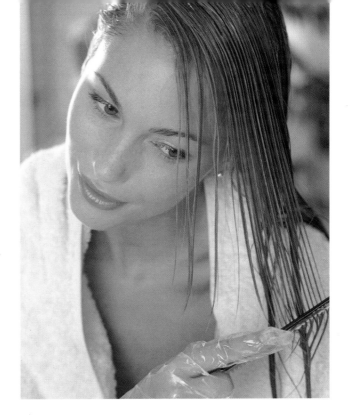

a few colour rules

■ **For a more natural effect,** keep within your own colour range, ie pale blonde rarely works with olive skin.

■ **Home colourants work best** if you have medium to dark hair and all you want to do is enrich the natural colour. You can avoid obvious regrowth by using a semi-permanent or wash-in, wash-out tint, both of which eventually just fade.

■ **When you want to vary your colour** by two shades or more, or cover more than 50 per cent grey, go professional. The reasons: the hairdresser can see all the way around your head, so the chances are it will be even and natural-looking. He or she can also gauge exactly which colour is right for your skin tone and make one up to suit you, rather than you having to choose from a limited selection of colours. In addition, salons can judge how porous your hair is, to ensure that you leave with the kind of colour you'd like. If in doubt, consult your hairdresser.

■ **When covering grey,** go for permanent colour but never more than two shades darker than your own natural colour. Lighter colours are more flattering with age: the skin tone also becomes paler as hair greys. Once grey, 'warmth in the hair helps pale skin look healthier,' says David Adams of natural beauty company Aveda. So if you were originally blonde, go lighter (honey, gold and fawn shades); if you were originally brunette, go warmer (auburn, copper and chestnut shades).

■ **Preserve and protect new colour** from the elements (sun, sea, water, pollution) and use haircare products specially formulated for coloured hair.

Always good to know …

■ Product build-up can interfere with the colouring process, so use a deep-cleansing detoxifying shampoo first for more even results.

■ Do a strand test. The thinner your hair, the less amount of time you need to achieve the colour you want, so try new colour out on a tiny bit of hair from the underneath layers first – just in case you don't like it.

■ If you are dyeing very long or very thick hair, you may need a second kit in case you run out of colour.

■ Use the colour as soon as you've prepared it: once chemicals oxidise they may give a different result from that shown on the box.

■ For hair that's longer than the chin: don't apply colour directly onto the ends – they're drier and more porous, and will absorb more colour than you probably want.

no shine

You only have to look at all the hair adverts to know that a glossy, shiny head of hair is the ideal. In comparison, dull hair simply looks dirty and out of condition. Luckily this is one of the easiest problems to rectify.

why hair doesn't shine

Dull hair only looks shiny when the protective coating (the cuticle) of each hair shaft lies flat, creating a smooth surface which reflects light beautifully. When cuticles are roughened through over-processing, overheating and poor conditioning, hair looks dull and out of condition.

The fastest way to polish up your hair is with a silk scarf. You may think this is an old wives' tale, but the silk particles really can help to smooth the hair's cuticles down so they lie flat, making hair look more glossy. Or you could sleep on a satin pillow, which will also help to smooth the hair cuticles, almost as if you've polished your hair.

how to care

Curly hair is less shiny than straight hair (and blonde hair is less shiny than that of brunettes and redheads) because straight hair reflects the light, while curls absorb it. Dry straight hair using a round radial brush to grip the hair well and give more control. Keep the nozzle of the hairdryer aiming down the hair shaft all the time you are drying, to ensure hair cuticles remain flat. Try setting wavy hair on velcro rollers to give a smoother finish.

tips for shiny hair

■ **Clean hair is more shiny.** City hair needs washing often, due to pollution and dust. Styling products lead to build-up which in turn leaves hair looking dull. Use a deep cleansing detox shampoo which is designed to cut down on residues.

■ **Shine serums and sprays** instantly smooth and varnish hair to reflect more light and look more shiny. Regularly apply conditioner. It not only adds gloss but coats and protects the hair from further damage caused by sun exposure and heated appliances.

■ **Deep conditioning treatments** can restore shine by smoothing and sealing the outer cuticle. Try a regular hot oil treatment: make your own by warming up a teacup of olive oil, comb through your hair and leave on for five minutes before rinsing thoroughly.

■ **Colour adds shine.** The warmer the colour, such as gold and red highlights, the shinier your hair will appear to be. Brunette and auburn hair look more shiny than blonde or grey hair, so add rich highlights to try to create the illusion of more light being reflected.

lack of volume

Call it limp, lank or greasy – this type of hair invariably goes flat after washing because it is thin and lacks body from the roots. But with careful styling and a bit of 'cheating' you can make your hair look thicker.

how to add body

The most effective way to add body to limp hair is by having a shampoo and set under a hooded hairdryer. This is because the extreme process of going from wet to dry, and from hot to cold, under the hood, sets the hair around big rollers, giving your hair extra lift just where it needs it – at the roots.

how to care

Thin hair tends to be greasy, so when you're looking after it yourself at home, it generally needs washing every day. Use a mild daily shampoo for frequent use. If you thoroughly wet your hair beforehand you will need to use less shampoo. Avoid 2-in-1 shampoo and conditioners (also called moisturising shampoos): these leave a residue in the hair that only weighs it down more. Apply a light conditioner to the ends only when your hair needs it.

Use styling products at the roots. The best formulation is a spray which is easy to direct precisely where you want it, and is quick drying. Volumisers coat hair to make it look and feel thicker by increasing the diameter of each individual hair shaft.

body building tips

■ **Semi-permanent and permanent hair dyes** penetrate and swell the hair shaft, so hair looks and feels thicker. The colour, too, can give the illusion of more body. Perming also swells the hair shaft and makes most hair types look thicker.

■ **A good cut can give the illusion of thicker hair.** A bob is probably the best style. For extra volume, graduate hair at the nape of the neck to lighten the load, coming forward to one length at the chin.

■ **The best way to add volume,** according to stylist Andrew Collinge, is to towel dry hair to remove excess moisture, then dry the roots off first by parting hair into sections and drying upside down, working in the opposite direction from the way hair grows.

■ **Change the way you blow-dry your hair.** Part your hair into sections, wrap the ends around a brush and lift the hair up and away in the opposite direction from which your hair grows. Direct the heat of the dryer to the roots, keeping it moving to avoid overheating the scalp.

dry ends

Only those with medium to long hair tend to suffer from dry ends. If we remember that long hair is well over three years old and has suffered abuse from hairdryers and UV light, it's easier to understand why the ends suffer.

what causes them?

Dry ends are largely self-inflicted, caused by over-zealous shampooing, not enough conditioner, harsh brushing, and too many heated styling appliances. All of which result in the end of the hair shaft splitting. However diet, stress and ill health are major factors too.

how to care

Use conditioner every time you wash your hair and apply to the ends, avoiding the roots which may be greasier. A deep-conditioning treatment once every two weeks will also help to keep hair softer, more supple, easier to brush and style, and so less vulnerable to damage.

Avoid washing dry hair every day; it doesn't need it. And when you do wash, dilute your shampoo: that same handful you always feel you need will still lather up, but you'll be using less detergent which will inevitably be less drying. Dry hair can get away with using heavier, moisturising, 2-in-1 shampoos which leave a fine film of conditioner on the strands. There's no need to apply shampoo to the ends – the action of rinsing will be sufficient to cleanse along the whole length of your hair.

It's a good idea to let your hair dry naturally if your style allows you to, as this will help to lock moisture in rather than drying it out.

Tips for dry ends

■ **If you want to blow-dry,** do it right: always keep the nozzle at least six inches away from your hair and constantly moving. Angle the heat downwards along the hair shaft to ensure that the cuticles lie flat and use the coolest heat possible.

■ **Avoid brushes with spiky, rough bristles** which catch hairs and snag them. Stick to a vent brush with widely spaced prongs, and never brush hair while it's wet.

■ **A regular trim is the only way to get rid of dry, split ends.** Trimming your hair also encourages healthier growth and thicker, blunt ends, so hair is less likely to split with regular care.

■ **Increase your intake of vitamin E** by eating more nuts and green vegetables. Alternatively, daily vitamin E oil capsules can help hair that is dry or brittle, says leading trichologist, Philip Kingsley.

■ **Tugging and pulling through tangles** causes breakage and split ends. An effective conditioner also acts as a detangler and should be combed through using a wide-tooth comb to help it slide through more easily.

frizz

Frizzy, flyaway hair is often the hardest hair to style because it is directly affected by the weather, giving it a will of its own when you least expect it. The trick is to keep it looking smooth and so more groomed.

why hair frizzes

Frizz is the result of too much moisture in the hair, which is why it tends to look worse in rainy or humid weather, or when you come out of the steam room. Frizzy hair tends to be quite dry and more porous, because the hair's natural protection is weak or damaged. The latest leave-in conditioners contain anti-humectants (water repellents) that seal the cuticles to prevent moisture from getting in the hair shaft, and stay there until you next shampoo. These can weigh hair down a little, but that can actually help to control frizz.

how to care

Choose heavier shampoos which contain proteins to coat each hair, making it more supple and helping to tame it down. You can control frizz by the way you dry your hair: either by leaving it to dry naturally, with a serum or pomade massaged in while it is still damp; or cool-dry hair smooth in sections using a hairdryer and starting with the underneath layers.

Apply styling products evenly through the hair. Whether you choose wax, serum or pomade, the trick is to warm the product in your hands first, which helps to spread it more evenly throughout your hair. Apply to underneath layers too, not just to the surface layers.

Tips for fighting frizz

■ **Avoid perming frizzy hair:** the process can make hair even harder to control afterwards.

■ **A regular cut can help to combat frizziness.** Coarse grey hair benefits most from a short, sharp cut. Long frizzy hair needs more graduation, cutting hair away from the face to allow less frizzy hair to show from underneath.

■ **Before swimming, apply a conditioner** – any will do – to your hair to act as a protective layer from the drying and bleaching effects of chlorine.

■ **Hair that's prone to frizz** will get better results from using a high-powered hairdryer, large brushes and heavier styling products such as waxes and pomades. All of these will help to smooth down frizzy and flyway hair.

■ **Carry a smoothing pomade or serum** around with you and apply as often as you think your hair needs calming down.

■ **When blow drying frizzy hair,** the roots should be dried off completely or else they'll begin to kink and frizz in seconds. Always aim the hairdryer down the hair shaft to close and smooth the cuticle.

haircare solutions

Help for those days when you can't do a thing with your hair.

■ **For a quick restart** when your hair won't behave, dampen down the outer layers with a water spray (such as a plant spray bottle filled with fresh water) or a ready-made styling spray. It allows you to restyle those all-important top layers in next to no time.

■ **'To create soft, smooth tumbling curls** use heated rollers – the bigger the roller, the looser the curl. Lightly spray dry hair with a spray gel or setting lotion, comb through, then wind small sections of hair around the rollers. Leave to cool, then remove each roller. Avoid brushing, simply apply a touch of serum to your fingers then coax around each curl to add gloss and definition.' suggests Charles Worthington.

■ **To maintain body all day long,** fluff hair with your fingers rather than brushing, which only tends to flatten. If your hair really does need a brush, do it from underneath with your head upside down, so you fluff instead of flatten.

■ **When you want to flip the ends out,** roll the hair under and around a brush and blow-dry it first. At the very last second, reverse the roll to flip out the curl.

■ **To curl the ends under** When your hair is completely dry, spray a round brush with light hairspray and use to roll the ends under. Before you unroll, heat with a hairdryer, then hit the cooling button to lock in the curl.

■ **For extra volume on the crown** Wait until your hair is almost dry, aim the dryer at the top of your head and rub your fingers in a back and forth motion at the roots, as if you're scratching your head.

■ **If you find velcro rollers don't stay in place** on their own, pin them in place to stop them from wobbling, otherwise you might end up with a kink in the hair around the roots. Blow-dry hair first, then place the rollers in dry hair to give a smoother wave, rather than tight curls.

■ **To cultivate curls,** use a diffuser attachment on your hairdryer and choose a medium heat setting on your hairdryer. It's kinder to hair because it styles quickly as it dries, but if it's too hot, hair will be fluffy, not curly, and dehydrated.

■ **If your hair is fine, weak and prone to split ends,** have a regular trim every six weeks to cut the splits out once they begin to occur, rather than waiting for them to split halfway up the length of the hair.

■ **If you suffer from combination hair** – greasy on the roots and dry at the ends – use a mild frequent wash shampoo daily, and resist the habit of running your hands through your hair, which only makes it oilier more quickly.

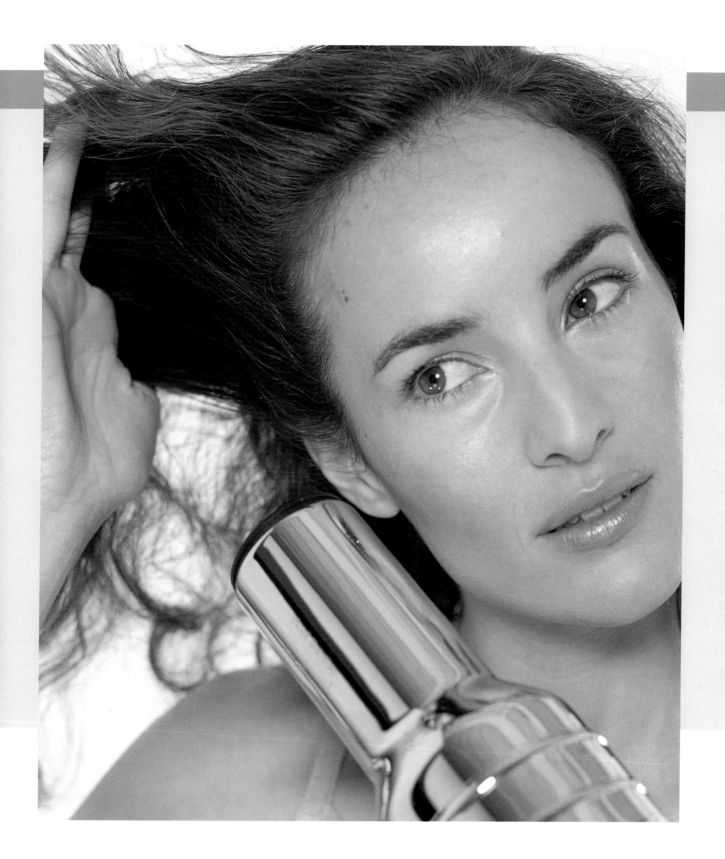

anti-ageing hairstyles

A good cut will be easy to manage if you know the right style for you [and your hair]. Leading hairdresser Neil Cornelius, at Micheljohn, suggests 5 styles that take years off your looks.

the classic bob 'This is one of the most flattering styles for all kinds of hair and face shapes,' says Neil. 'You can vary the length of the bob depending on how round or thin your face is, and if you have jowls, a longer length bob like Twiggy's is more age-defying than cutting it shorter and revealing all. Only avoid a bob if you have very curly hair as it tends to lose the shape and can look more old-fashioned than stylish and modern.'

a graduated bob 'This has shaping around the front to soften the geometric shape we associate with a more classic bob. Adding a light fringe or feathering at the sides helps to create softness which is more flattering with age. If in doubt, always start with a classic bob as a base to begin with, and then you can layer into it afterwards to vary the shape and make it softer.'

add a fringe 'Quite often women add a fringe to their style to cover up frown lines on the forehead. The only problem is that the deeper the frowns become, the thicker the fringe seems to be, and then the whole balance of the face is lost. Avoid a heavy fringe: keep it light and chop into it to create a more flattering, feathered effect. It will still hide frown lines, but the overall effect is much more rejuvenating.'

long layered hair 'I think it's a myth that women past a certain age shouldn't have long hair,' says Neil. 'What matters most is its condition and how well the hair is looked after.' The trick to having flattering long hair is styling it to 'shape' the front (not layering it, which thins hair too much) so that you lose that hippie 'curtain of hair' which is less attractive.

shorter layered, feathered styles 'These frame the face and have a gamine appeal which suits most faces, particularly those with petite features such as actress Dame Judi Dench. Feathering around the hairline is gentler and more forgiving than having hair scraped or slicked back severely, and a halo of hair softens age and bony features. Layers can be coaxed away from the scalp to conceal roots and give the illusion of more body to fine, thinning hair.'

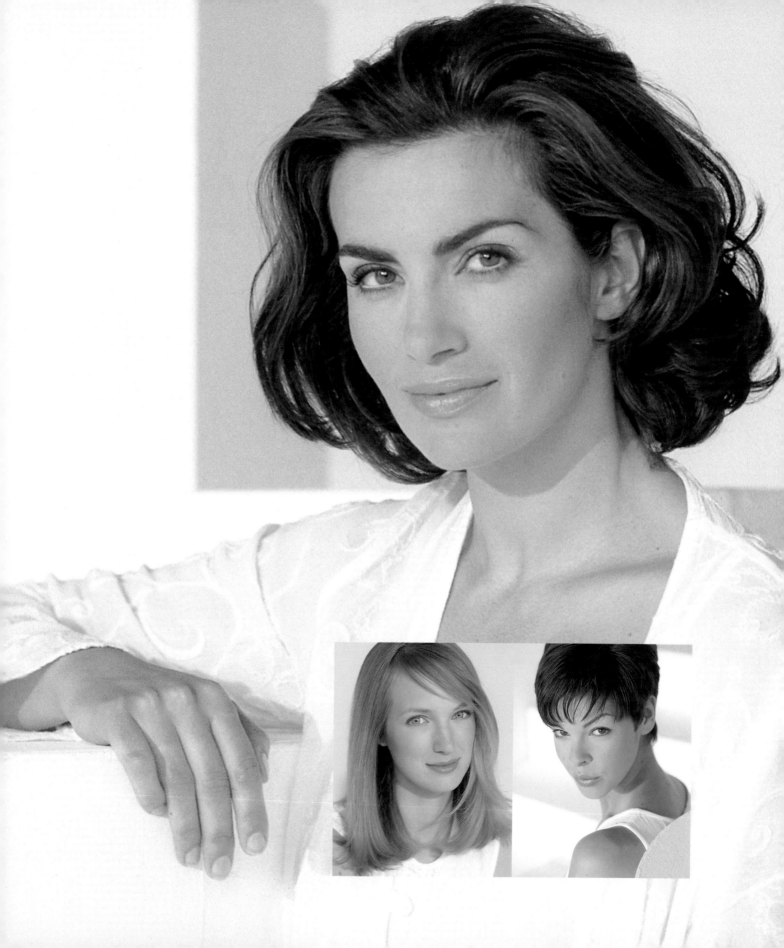

salon speak

How can you translate what you want into a hairstyle you like, and make it an experience worth going back to the salon for again and again? Here's how to get salon savvy and find a look you love.

getting the best cut

■ **Have a consultation first.** A consultation should be free. Go when your hair is looking its most natural and dress the way you like to look. Communication starts before you even say a word: hairdressers often make up their mind about you simply from the way you dress.

■ **Take a few photos,** especially if you are having your hair cut by someone new. It gives you both something concrete to refer back to – in terms of length, volume, shape – if communication is becoming a problem.

■ **Decide what you want before you go** – you'll be less likely to be swayed by a wilful stylist doing just what he wants. Be realistic about the look you're after. A cute 'Cameron Diaz' just might not be the one for you. And be honest about how much time you really spend on your hair. There's no point going for a look that takes hours to perfect when you should have been out of the door an hour ago.

■ **Look at the stylist.** Do you like her hair? If you do, don't book her – book the one who cut it. Take a look around the salon. Is it buzzing with life or seriously conservative? 'If you don't see a lot of young people coming in, it means the salon is not modern enough and moving forward,' says Charles Worthington. 'If the shop and your stylist are really busy, you can feel more confident.'

■ **Go by word of mouth:** it is still one of the best ways to find a stylist.

how much should I tip?

'Hairdressing is a tipping profession,' says Clive Lever at Michaeljohn, 'and the juniors are on such a small wage, they pretty much depend upon it.' But remember that it's a gratuity, you're not obliged to pay, so only give something (10–15 per cent is the norm) if you're suitably pleased with the job.' The problem is that by the time you've had a shampoo, cut, colour, another shampoo (by another junior) then a final blow-dry, you'll have doubled your bill as you'd have to tip everyone! The general rule is tip the junior first (they need it more), and if you feel generous, tip the stylist then the owner.

not happy?

If you are unhappy with the results, knowing your rights makes it much easier to complain. Hopefully if you've taken all the precautions above, you've minimised any chances of not liking your hair, but if problems do still arise, communication is vital, so speak up there and then. As a guide: if you have a problem with a junior or the receptionist, tell the stylist. If it's about the cut or colour, talk to the stylist calmly but directly. Don't leave dissatisfied. Any decent salon will remedy the situation – after all, you are a walking advertisement for the salon. If you've washed it yourself and it's not working for you; the fringe is too heavy, the sides are still too long – call them, don't wait more than a week. They should offer you a complimentary cut to rectify it.

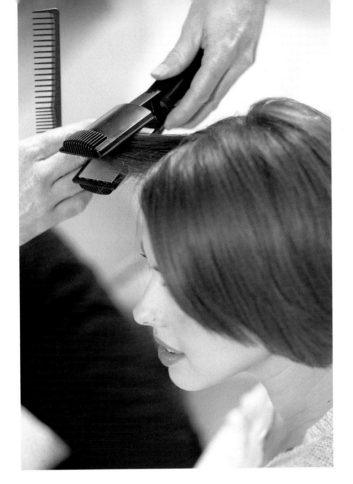

How to help the hairdresser

■ **Don't hold anything back.** For example, if you've had colour on your hair already, are on medication or pregnant, the colour may come out differently than expected. A good salon will do a strand test first but, if in doubt, now's the time to speak.

■ **Show the stylist some photos and explain exactly what you like about them.** Most hairdressers prefer clients to provide some solid guidance rather than risk misunderstanding.

Gift of the gab

Hairdressers have their own unique 'hair speak' – special words and phrases they've dreamed up to make a quick snip sound very technical! Memorise these and you'll sound like a pro yourself.

■ **Blunt cut:** creating a one-layer, straight, solid edge.

■ **Chipping (also called point cut):** softening the ends of the hair, especially a fringe, by pointing the scissors into the ends rather than cutting across, to give better texture.

■ **Feathering (also called razor cutting):** using a razor or sharp scissors to add softness and texture, and to reduce thickness.

■ **Freehand:** creating a style by working with the hair's natural texture and wave.

■ **Graduated layers:** layering from short to long, such as around the face from fringe to shoulders.

■ **Slide cutting:** sliding the scissors down the hair length, especially on the hair around the face, to give a softer and more flattering edge.

■ **Texturising:** softening a cut by removing any hard lines and blunt edges with a freehand.

■ **Undercutting:** leaving long layers on top and short layers underneath. Very stylish right now and great for giving texture to flat hair.

your mind

well-being is not just about

eating better, exercising

more, looking after your body

or feeling good about the

way you look. It's also about

finding balance, health,

happiness and contentment

in all areas of your life

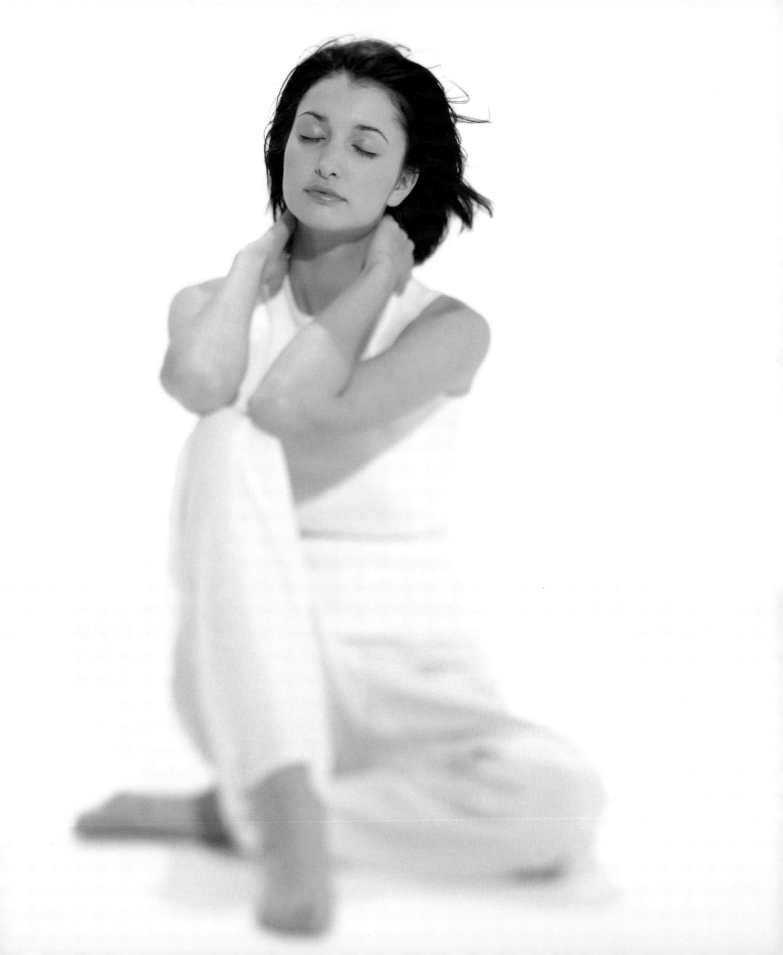

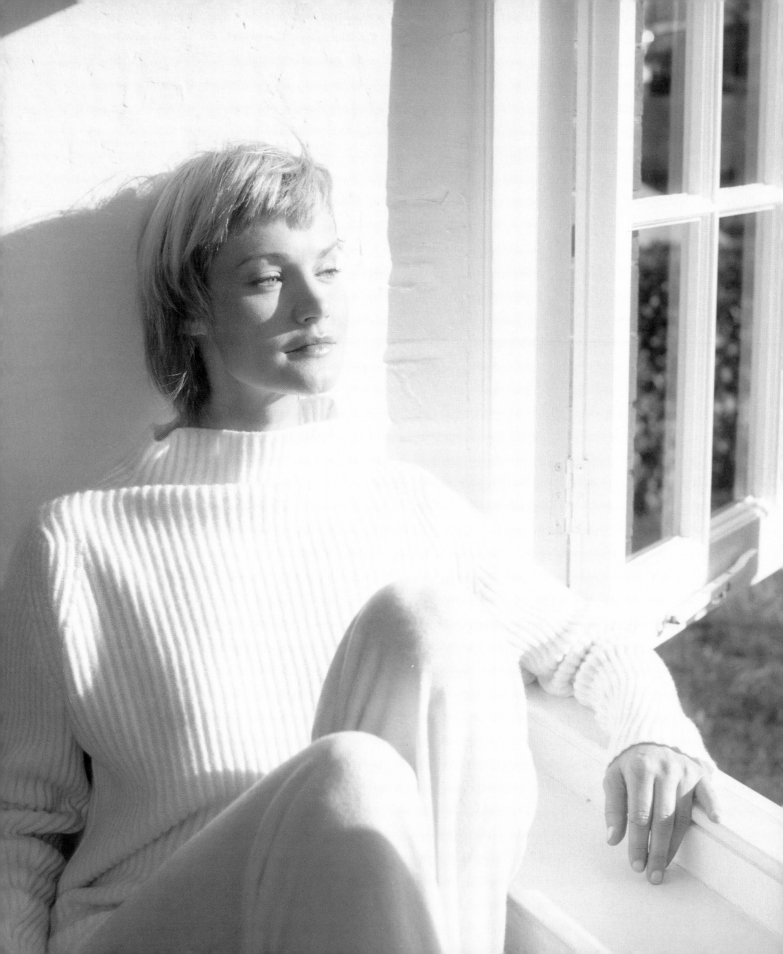

how and why your mind ages

what's going on

We are what we believe ourselves to be. If we don't believe in ourselves, why should anyone else? Teach your mind to work for you instead of against you for greater inner strength.

your mind over matter

How you think has a direct effect on the way you look and feel. The power of the mind is exceptional. Doctors and psychologists have long believed that stress can make illnesses worse, and when you are depressed or have a major setback in life – such as losing your job, bereavement or divorce – you are much more likely to go down with a bug. Being in a positive state of mind, however, has been shown to have a powerful uplifting effect on your body.

use it or lose it

Ageing should be viewed as a process of maturation, not deterioration. Keep your brain busy and lively and you guarantee enjoying an active old age; lose it and you cease to be active in both mind and body. So exercise your brain. Play games that make you think, read books that challenge you, listen to music.

feed your brain

Our brains are affected by the same processes that contribute to overall aging, so how well we have taken care of ourselves throughout our lives affects not only our general health, but also our mental function. The brain is a ravenous consumer of glucose and oxygen, both of which are supplied by the blood. If your heart is weakened by years of inactivity or if your arteries are clogged with cholesterol, then your memory and mental functioning will be impaired. As with the rest of your body, increasing the amount of antioxidants in your diet will help to protect vital cells, including those in the brain, from free radical damage.

Ginkgo biloba contains flavonoids, potent antioxidants. It helps to improve circulation and delivery of oxygen and nutrients to the brain and can also be helpful in combating memory loss, improving mental function, and alleviating depression, dizziness, ringing in the ears and headaches. Another herb for improving mental function is ginseng. This is an adaptogen, which improves the body's ability to adapt to a broad range of physical and biochemical conditions and stressors.

positive mind and body tips

Great ideas to help keep you thinking – and thereby looking – younger.

■ **'Develop a more positive approach to your health.** Being a hypochondriac is a negative attitude to life and can lead to the taking of too many unnecessary drugs.' Leading Chinese herbalist Michael McIntyre.

■ **'Taking extra vitamins** won't give you any more energy, unless you are already deficient to begin with. However, women of childbearing age, vegetarians, chronic dieters and endurance exercisers are most likely to be deficient in one or more vital vitamins or minerals. In these cases it's a good idea to take a multivitamin with iron to keep energy soaring.' Nutritionist Ann Louise Gittleman.

■ **Try age therapy.** Play at doing teenage things, such as listening to the kind of music you enjoyed back then.

■ **'Increase your movement** and total body workout. Children are eternal optimists. They never stop, and a run across a playground is for them a total body workout. But as adults we just seem to come to a standstill.' Top American dermatologist Karen Burke,

■ **Recharge your batteries.** You can't make skin immortal, but you can make it think it's younger than it really is.' Astrologer Shelley von Strunckel.

■ **'Relax.** Get beyond ageing. Worrying about it will only accelerate the process.' Teresa Hale of London complementary health centre, The Hale Clinic.

■ **Get a pet.** Research suggests that rhythmical stroking is relaxing and soothing and can help prevent heart attacks. Stroking a dog, cat or other pet can therefore really help you live longer.

■ **Deep breathing** is the best way for you to calm your whole body down when you feel tense and under pressure. Try this breathing exercise: sit upright in a comfortable chair, with your hands resting on your stomach. Breathe in fully, count to two, then breathe out for a count of six at the same rate. Be aware of your hands rising and falling. Repeat 12 times.

■ **Just do it.** Procrastination is simply a waste of your valuable time. If there's something new you want to learn – for example, ballooning, hang-gliding, bungey jumping or whatever – don't just think about it and do nothing, which will bring you down. Work out the how, when, where and just go for it.

■ **'People who deal in sunshine** are the ones who draw the crowds. They always do more business than those who peddle clouds.' Anon.

■ **Misery is catching.** Make an audio tape of your own conversation for an hour or two and play it back. You might be surprised at the level of negativity, cynicism and personal put-downs you use. Remember, it's in your power to be miserable or to be joyous. Perhaps people around you have an effect. Make it your plan to surround yourself with happy, positive people, and to be specially positive around those who moan. You – and they – will benefit hugely.

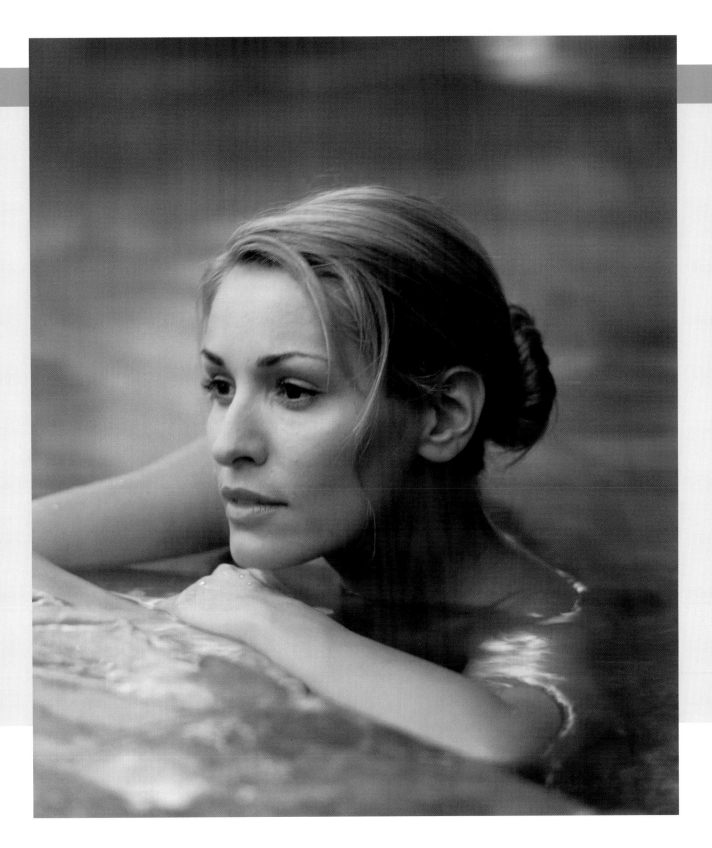

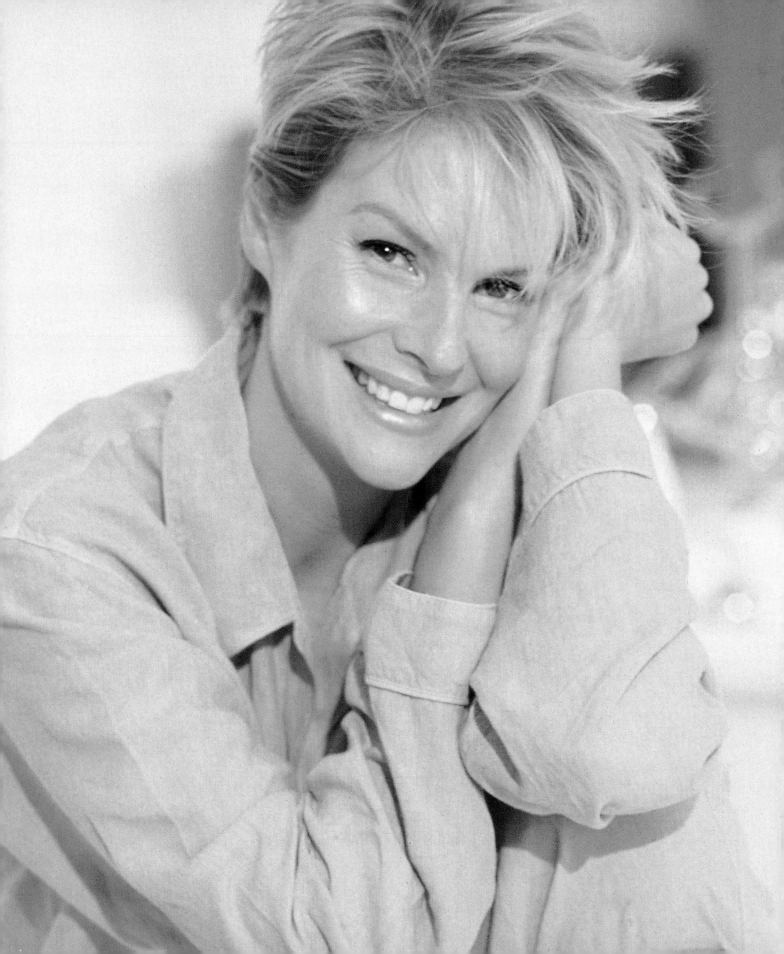

daily mind and body requirements

mind, body, spirit

Adopt a more harmonious lifestyle, with peaceful moments for reflection. Seek out ways to stop the clock and unwind for a few moments each day, and you will find rejuvenation.

promote well-being

Your mind, body and spirit are inextricably linked together. While you may accept that your body will operate on auto-pilot and perform at a certain level regardless of your lifestyle choices, there's no denying that it will serve you better if it is nurtured, loved and appreciated. To promote well-being of the mind, body and spirit – and so encourage happiness, longevity and inner radiance – aim to include some of the following mental and physical activities in your life.

Practise deep breathing or yoga, meditation, Pilates or T'ai Chi. Try and incorporate some form of daily massage into your life, and treat yourself to aromatherapy. Aerobic exercise will get the blood circulating: aim for 20 minutes until you begin to perspire. Practise inner and outer cleansing and detoxification; set positive goals and make regular positive affirmations to yourself.

Make your mind a sanctuary: a place where you can find peace and tranquillity when you need it. Take time to reflect on your emotions, to look within yourself and discover a new sense of self just when you need it most.

relax your body

Tension runs throughout the body, any time of the day. Without realising it, you may grit your teeth for control in times of anger, clench the steering wheel, hunch your shoulders and screw up your eyes in deep concentration. Yet relax your muscles, and you de-stress your mind, body and spirit in one. Learn to love and respect your body by giving it the attention it deserves and it will reward you in the long run.

free your spirit

Often when you feel overloaded by every aspect of your life, you need to take a step back from the daily routine and simply switch off. A positive outlook frees the mind, body and spirit, but it is only by letting go that you can see beyond the obstacles that are placed before you. Let the joy of living come into your life each day and you will feel renewed and energised once more. To be spirited, you need spirit. Seek and find your true sense of worth, so that you can rekindle your spirit and enliven your soul.

self belief

The 'midlife crisis' is fast becoming a concern for women. It may be that you gave up a career to have children and 20 years later, now that they've grown up and left home, you find you've lost your sense of self. Perhaps you're going through a divorce and have lost the confidence in yourself to feel able to start all over again, or maybe you've followed a lifelong career, chosen not to have a family, and suddenly find yourself made redundant. Self-worth is crucial. Belief in yourself is everything, because if you don't believe in yourself, why should anyone else?

positive power

Having a negative attitude to life puts you on the road to premature ageing, fast. Positive thinking is being able to use your thoughts and feelings to find a way forward, instead of being held back by attitudes and beliefs. Here are some ideas to help you:

■ **Recognise your strengths** When you are faced with a problem, remember the things you are good at instead of focusing on the difficult things. This way you are using more of the resources needed to solve the problem.

■ **Use flexible thinking** Have you tried to solve a similar problem in the past? Thinking flexibly means seeing the problem from lots of different angles, which increases the possibility of finding a realistic solution.

■ **Set positive goals** Aim for what you want to gain, not what you want to lose. So set your goal as 'I want to become fit and healthy', rather than 'I want to lose weight'.

■ **Start with small, achievable goals** Mountains are daunting: small steps are encouraging. So having set yourself an overall target, break it down into the steps you need to take to achieve your goal. As the Chinese proverb says: 'A journey of 1,000 miles starts with one step.' And give yourself a reward at stages along the way.

■ **Become aware of the things you say to yourself** Over the years we acquire beliefs about ourselves – often from other people – such as, 'I am a failure' or 'I have no willpower'. Like all generalisations they are often not true and can be successfully challenged and replaced by positive self-statements.

what is stress?

We all need a certain amount of stress in our lives. It's the power behind much creative thought, action and achievement. But when it becomes too much, we can feel overwhelmed, developing symptoms such as insomnia, overworking, eating or drinking too much, depression and irritability. These in turn lead to physical and mental exhaustion.

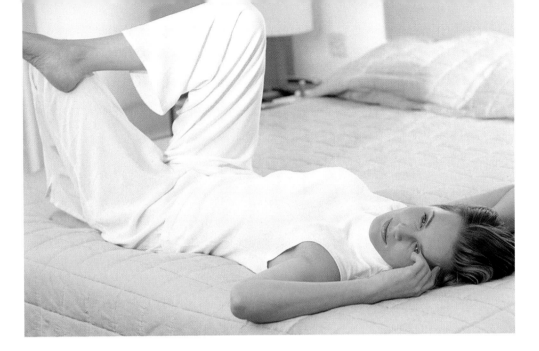

10 ways to keep calm

■ **This yoga position is very relaxing** and good for your back. Get down on the floor on your hands and knees, then stretch your arms right out in front of you until your forehead rests on the floor too. Breathe in slowly, and then out.

■ **Sit comfortably in a chair** and lift your shoulders right up to your ears. Hold for a few seconds, then lower again. Repeat three to four times. Then, to help free the neck, rock your head gently from side to side.

■ **Put two to three drops of balancing geranium essential oil** in a bowl with a little warm water and leave it to diffuse, scenting the air.

■ **Lie down flat and still,** and focus on your breathing, telling yourself that you feel warm and peaceful. Be aware of the weight of your body becoming heavier and heavier, limb by limb, until you feel unable to move. Concentrate on your breathing for five minutes, then when you are ready, wiggle your toes and fingers, open your eyes and get up slowly.

■ **Sit cross-legged with your back supported** by a sofa or chair. Close your eyes, and place one hand on your abdomen, below the ribs, and the other on your chest. Breathe in slowly through your nose, and concentrate on moving only the lower hand. Breathe quietly and calmly for 10 minutes.

■ **We hold a lot of tension in the jaw without realising.** Relax for a few moments and chew something slowly to relieve tension.

■ **Listen to a piece of your favourite music** to help you to relax.

■ **Breathe in as slowly as you can** (try to get to the count of 10), then breathe out equally slowly. It's a quick way to calm down, and it works.

■ **Take a brisk walk** in the fresh air for 10–20 minutes.

■ **Laugh.** Put on a favourite comedy video. Sit back, relax and enjoy it.

Treat yourself

■ **Buy flowers** for yourself ... instead of for everyone else.

■ **Visit a health spa**, and pamper yourself from top to toe.

■ **Learn something new** Take classes in salsa, a language, or learn to play an instrument

■ **Read that book** you've had on your shelves for so long.

■ **Start to paint** Be more creative with your time.

stress

Stress is ageing, adding years to your skin and multiplying your chances of developing a chronic illness. Learning to deal with it head-on through relaxation techniques will arm you with the power to overcome any obstacle.

time to relax

Deep breathing, stress therapy, positive thinking and laughter therapy are all effective methods of relaxation that you can build into your everyday life. Put aside 10–20 minutes for yourself every day to practise some form of relaxation.

yoga

This ancient art combines relaxation and exercise for both mind and body. It is considered to be an ideal way to reduce stress levels and restore the natural equilibrium of your body. The postures (or *Asanas*) are all gentle stretches which improve balance, strength and flexibility, coupled with correct breathing techniques. They work on the entire body including the internal organs, which are massaged by specific movements. There are a number of different yoga techniques, so the safest way to practise it is with a fully qualified instructor.

aquatherapy

Also known as hydrotherapy. Water is a natural tranquilliser that soothes the emotions. It makes our spirits as buoyant as our bodies, and is the best escape from the weight of gravity and the pressures of the world. The potential of mind–water therapy has not been fully explored, but British psychiatrists have been treating emotionally disturbed patients 'aquatically', by adding the sound of waves and the smell of the sea in sessions.

In France, free-floating in a pool is used to treat stress: sufferers strap on a body float, lie back and listen to ethereal music as they relax. Flotation tanks involve lying in silence in a dark tank, floating in just a few inches of extremely salty, and buoyant, water. A half-hour float can feel as good as a full eight hours' sleep as your brain switches over to more relaxing theta wave patterns. (These patterns occur in the early stages of sleep, when the brain is still receptive to outside influences but your body is rested.)

t'ai chi

A form of mental and physical exercise that gives a sense of inner calm. Practitioners credit it with powers such as giving you the ability to complete projects at work without stress, overcome personal trauma or simply to cope with the children and the housework. Many of the exercises in T'ai chi are based on the graceful movements of animals, and have equally poetic names such as 'the white crane spreads its wings' and 'the white ape presents fruit'. Each movement is full of energy and power while being completely relaxed.

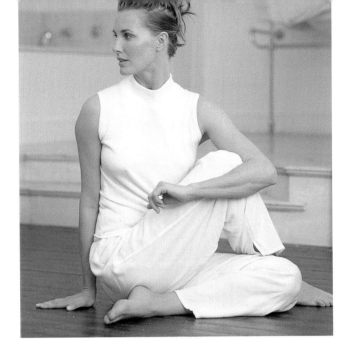

meditation

An ideal antidote to stress, meditation has been found to slow down the body's metabolism, heart rate and breathing, as well as lower blood pressure, boost the immune system, reduce muscle tension and ease aches and pains. The ultimate mind, body and soul therapy, it is now used to treat a variety of stress-related conditions including palpitations, depression and anxiety, insomnia, stuttering and headaches. The idea is to clear your mind of its constant daily noise and interruptions and just concentrate on one single thing in order to find peace and tranquillity.

There are several different types of meditation. Transcendental Meditation (TM) involves repeating a mantra (a word of phrase given to you by a TM teacher). Autogenic training uses mental exercises designed to help you switch stress off and switch relaxation systems on whenever you need them.

Mindfulness concentrates on a single activity to heighten awareness, such as eating, breathing or listening, and Zen meditation uses mind puzzles called 'koans' to help you focus your mind.

laughter therapy

Laughter is deeply therapeutic, and goes way beyond just raising a smile. It relaxes muscles, relieves tiredness, improves circulation and boosts the immune system by triggering the release of the antibody immunoglobulin A. Laughter supports the most basic theory of well-being: if something feels good, it will be good for you.

visualisation

The art of relaxation through mental imagery. While you are practising deep breathing, close your eyes and focus your mind on a happy, peaceful place you've been to. Now imagine yourself there again. Happiness is truly the most positive therapy imaginable.

Relax your mind and body

Just a few quiet minutes a day can help you to train your mind to relax your body. Unplug the phone and put earplugs in if necessary. Create peace in your environment to find peace within.

- **Sit quietly in a comfortable position.**
- **Relax your muscles (if you find this hard to do, focus on one limb at a time).**
- **Pick a focus word or image, such as 'calm' or 'love', or concentrate on your breathing.**
- **Breathe slowly and naturally and repeat the chosen word as you breathe out.**
- **If other thoughts intrude, simply say 'Oh well', and carry on repeating your word.**
- **Continue for about 20 minutes.**

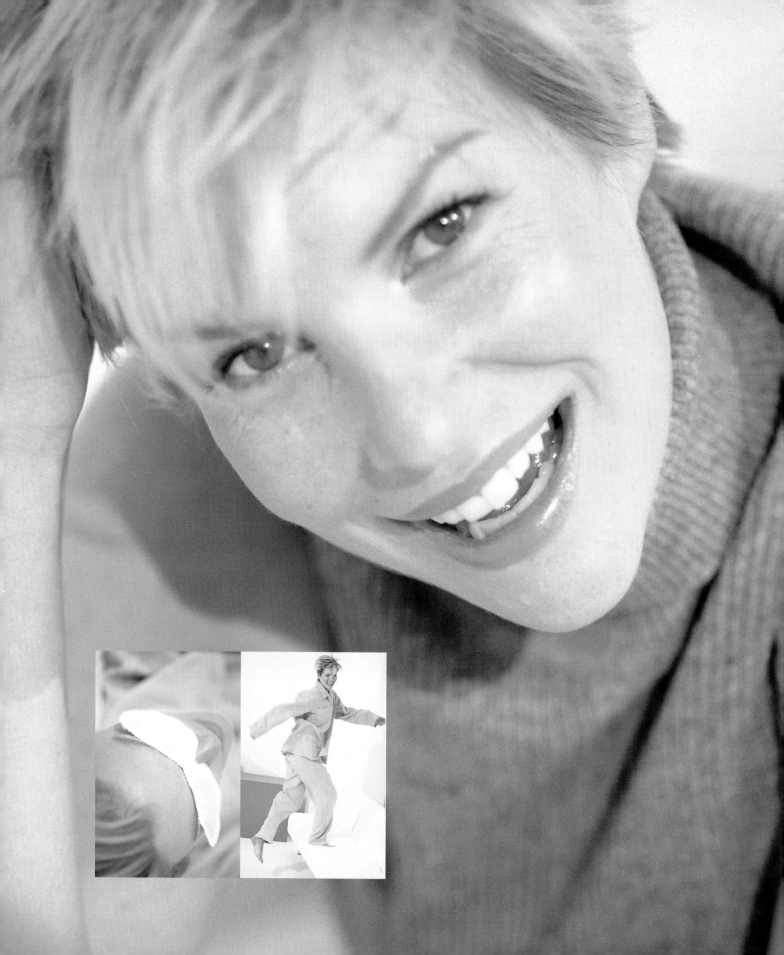

anti-ageing mind workout

Revitalise your mind and body in one go with Daoyin, the ancient Chinese exercise that uses breathing techniques and simple movements to promote tranquillity and relaxation.

We know that aerobic exercise (such as walking, running, swimming, cycling, tennis and squash) increases blood flow and volume, strengthens heart and lungs, and lowers your resting heart rate, all of which help you to accomplish your daily activities with far less physical effort and fatigue. But the best regime you can follow is a combination of aerobic and deep breathing exercise.

Universally practised for centuries in the East, and fast becoming increasingly popular in the West, many rebalancing, deep breathing exercises such as yoga and T'ai chi offer energising effects for your body...and your mind. Yoga originates from India and offers a wide range of health-giving and rejuvenating properties to anyone of any age and fitness level. The word 'yoga', translated from Sanskrit, means 'union', and literally represents a joining of the body and mind as one.

T'ai chi originates from China and means 'wholeness'. It is based on the Eastern belief that illness is due to emotional disturbance that usually comes from an imbalance in the flow of energy, or Qi (pronounced 'chee') through the body.

All about Daoyin

Daoyin (Daoyin Yangsheng Gong) is one of the oldest known and most researched systems of health training in China, but is still little known in the UK. It is an exercise régime that emphasises deep relaxation and energises body and mind through slow, tranquil, twisting movements, thereby improving body co-ordination, balance, stress levels, breathing awareness and quality of sleep.

'As well as being a great supplement to a busy lifestyle,' says Simon Watson, British Martial Arts champion and Daoyin instructor, 'Daoyin has also been used for its healing powers for disorders connected with the heart, circulation, and nervous system, as well as muscular injuries and asthma.' It is mind-absorbing, rather than physically exhausting or stressful, and consists of a series of slow continuous movements designed to relax and develop the whole body. The aim of the carefully structured movements is to improve posture and build up the body's internal strength and stamina.

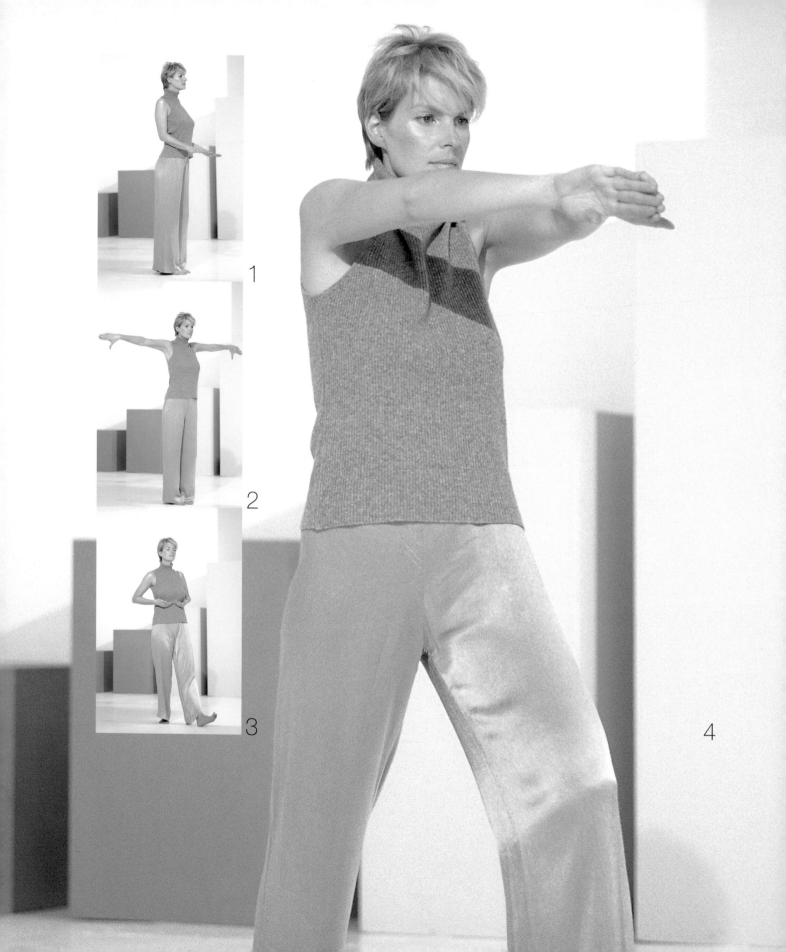

1

2

3

4

Starting position Start by standing straight, feet together, knees relaxed and slightly bent, hands by sides. Imagine you are facing the 12 o'clock position. The whole exercise is one complete movement without any pause – move slowly and gently into each position.

Turn to the left Breathing in, turn your upper body from the waist to the left, to 10:30 and bring your arms to the position shown [1] with palms down. Bend your wrist so the backs of the hands face out in front of you, then circle your arms out to the sides, keeping the backs of your hands facing forwards so the arms feel as if they are twisting and stretching.

Circle the arms From the position shown [2] follow the movement through a complete circle, bringing the hands back to back, stretched out in front of you at chest height. This should emphasise the twist.

Turn to the right Move your weight on to your right foot and place your left heel out at 10:30, leaving the toes raised [3]. Turn the upper body back to the right to face 12:00 as you sweep the hands back towards you, backs of hands still together, then 'wiping' the tummy with the backs of the hands and turning the palms up under the bust. Then with the elbows remaining close to your sides, bring the hands behind your back, palms facing each other.

Transfer your weight Breathe out, bringing the arms out from behind you in a wide circle back to position 2 and through to position 4 as you transfer your weight over onto your left foot. Bend the knee slightly as you bring your hands down on to your left thigh, one hand on top of the other. Don't raise the rear foot. Hold this position for a count of three.

Return to starting position Breathe in. Bring the hands inwards as you 'sit back' on to the right foot, raising the front toes. The backs of the hands should rub against the tummy one more time with the palms finally turning upwards. Breathe out and return to the starting position. Perform the whole movement three times on the left side, then repeat three times on the right side, switching your weight over to the right side and turning the upper body to 1.30 when required.

What you need

- Wear loose, comfortable clothing that doesn't constrict your movements, and bare feet or socks on a non-slippery floor.
- Choose a gentle relaxation tape (such as *Temple in the Forest* by David Naegle) that will help you to focus on your movements without being too intrusive and interfering with your concentration.

glossary

Allergens is a term given to any ingredients known to cause an allergic reaction. Classic examples are PABA (which used to be found in sunscreens),formaldehyde and toluene.

Alpha hydroxy acids (AHAs) loosen dead skin so that it sheds to reveal a fresher, smoother complexion. Research shows that AHAs can also help your skin retain more moisture and speed up cell renewal. Products containing AHA can't make skin more taut or get rid of wrinkles, but can make it look clearer and radiant instantly. Some AHAs have been known to trigger skin problems in people that have fair or sensitive skin. Citric, glycolic, lactic and malic acids are examples of AHAs.

Antioxidants are mostly vitamins – beta-carotene (the precursor to vitamin A), C and E – plus zinc, and a few plants such as green tea and gingko biloba. Including them in your diet or taking them as supplements gives the best natural protection from the ageing effects of damage from free radicals (see F). Antioxidants are often used in skincare and suncare products to provide additional environmental protection.

Aromatherapy is a treatment which uses pure extracts of aromatic plants and flowers (such as lavender, rose and camomile), called pure essential oils, to heal common ailments and restore emotional balance. These oils enter the system via the bloodstream and stimulate receptors in the nose. This in turn relays messages to the limbic centre of the brain which controls all our emotions and feelings. Pure essential oils can be used in carrier oils for massage, diluted in the bath or diffused in the air using a vaporiser, or with steam.

Benzol peroxide is an anti-bacterial agent traditionally used in acne and spot treatments. It attacks the symptoms but not the cause. Known side effects include irritations and excessive dryness.

Beta-carotene is an important anti-ageing antioxidant vitamin found in carotenoid foods (usually red and green foods such as apricots, carrots, peppers, sweet potatoes and leafy vegetables) and is the precursor to vitamin A: ie the body naturally converts beta-carotene into vitamin A.

Beta-hydroxy acids (BHAs) behave like AHAs, brightening the skin and adding radiance by exfoliating dead skin cells. The most common BHA is salicylic acid (see S) which dermatologists often prefer because it rarely causes irritations, and is a gentle substitute for AHAs.

Bioflavonoids, known as flavones or citrus salts, are the main source of red and blue pigment in fruit (think blackcurrants, blueberries, cherries and papaya). With their anti-inflammatory properties, they are believed to help with fluid retention, varicose veins, allergies, reducing high blood pressure and relieving fatigue. Another great antioxidant, they help to protect the body from free radical damage, and can help to boost skin suppleness.

Calendula is the trendy name to call it – mere marigold is its name. An age-old ingredient known for its ability to strengthen, soothe and heal, it contains natural steroid substances called sterols and is suitable for dry or cracked skin and eczema.

Cellulite is the term given to the dimpled, orange-peel look which the majority of women get on their thighs and bottom, and sometimes on the backs of arms. Women of all shapes and sizes and levels of fitness get it, and on the whole men do not. The cause is not known, but the theory is that it relates directly to the level of the female hormone oestrogen. Some experts believe that cellulite is a sign of long-term imbalances within the body, and can be improved by cutting down on fat and sugar, drinking more water to flush out toxins, and boosting the circulation and the lymphatic system with regular exercise and manual massage.

Ceramides are naturally occurring lipids (or oils) found in the skin, which retain extra moisture. Artificial ceramides have been developed to help boost natural moisture levels in the skin.

Collagen is a vital skin protein which determines how supple, smooth and elastic skin is. Young skin has closely knitted collagen fibres, but age and free-radical damage from the sun and pollution cause these fibres to break down and skin loses its suppleness. Although it is added to skincare creams, collagen cannot be absorbed into the skin. Instead it acts as humectant, attracting water to the skin's surface.

Comedogenic signifies that a skin or make-up product is likely to cause comedones (or blackheads) on the skin. A 'non-comedogenic' product won't cause blackheads.

Dehydration occurs when the body doesn't have enough water reserves. It can be caused by illness, hormone levels, weather, central heating, air conditioning, anxiety and stress. Signs of dehydration can be seen on the skin first, as water is directed to vital internal organs. Even oily and combination skins can become dehydrated.

Detoxification literally means removing the toxins from your body – a spring clean from the inside out. A toxic overload results from a long list of daily poisons, such as alcohol, sugar, coffee, food additives, pesticides and pollution, and skin, hair

and nails are the first areas to show the signs. Health experts recommend detoxing for a couple of days a month, by drinking plenty of mineral water, avoiding wheat and dairy foods, and practising deep breathing exercises to calm and relax the system.

Dihydroxyacetone (DHA) is the main ingredient used in most self-tanning products. It gives skin the fake tan colour and is considered safe as it only tints the top layers of the skin, which is why colour only lasts up to five days.

Dry skin-brushing is an intense form of body exfoliation. As well as smoothing skin and boosting circulation, it is an invaluable part of detoxification, helping to stimulate lymphatic drainage and eliminate up to 30 per cent of the body's wastes. It should be done before showering, on dry skin with a soft-bristled brush. Using sweeping movements, work over the body from the soles of your feet towards the heart.

Echinacea is well known for boosting our immune system, and has excellent anti-inflammatory properties too, as well as helping to stimulate cellular repair at the same time.

Elastin, like collagen, is a protein which forms a vital part of the skin's connective tissue.

Electrolysis is a permanent method of hair removal using a fine needle which kills the hair at the follicle. It should be carried out by a qualified beauty therapist in a salon. It is ideal for small areas, such as the upper lip, chin and brows.

Enzymes are natural proteins and currently the hottest thing in skincare technology. Skin naturally contains 'good' and 'bad' enzymes. By harnessing beneficial enzymes and stopping the production of harmful ones, in theory skin should become better able to protect itself.

Essential fatty acids (EFAs) are natural oils (Omega 6 and Omega 3) essential for skin health, suppleness and long term moisture levels. GLA (Omega 6) is an EFA found mainly in evening primrose oil, Linolenic acid (Omega 3) is an EFA mainly found in flaxseed oil.

Exfoliation is the action of removing dead cells from the surface of the skin to make skin appear brighter and more radiant. It also helps to speed up a sluggish natural cell renewal cycle, which slows down naturally with age.

Free radicals are highly unstable molecules which are created naturally through oxidation, which leads to the breakdown of all living cells. They occur especially when we're put under daily stress from the sun, pollution, smoke, and even our emotions. In the skin, free radicals attack the DNA and our skin's natural repair mechanism. Young skin has enough protective power to neutralise free radicals. But as we age, our defences are weakened and free radical damage leads to the breakdown in collagen and elastin, leading to sagging skin and wrinkles.

Gamma-linolenic acid (GLA) is an essential fatty acid found mainly in evening primrose oil and starflower oil. It is vital for keeping the skin smooth and supple from within.

Ginkgo biloba has been found to have powerful anti-oxidant properties which help protect the body from oxidative damage to the body tissues (including your skin) caused by daily living and environmental exposure. Studies also show that ginkgo leaves help to strengthen the capillary walls, have a moisturising effect, are anti-inflammatory and stimulate the micro-circulation.

Ginger is without doubt a 'hot' ingredient right now! Highly stimulating and loved for its spicy aroma and the warming effect on the body, it boosts the circulation and remedies aches and pains.

Ginseng is the world's most famous herbal. Throughout the Orient it is valued as much as gold and its power was first discovered centuries ago, when chewing on the ginseng root was found to revive flagging spirits. Today, science has confirmed that it improves physical endurance and concentration.

Grapeseed extract is a natural anti-fungal, anti-viral treatment for many infections, including sore throats and cystitis. Now the beauty industry is using it as a highly effective antioxidant, because it is rich in polyphenols.

Green tea is one of the most powerful antioxidants and is found in almost every hot new skincare product at the moment, because it helps to inhibit the release of free radicals in the skin which cause premature ageing. The latest research has shown that green tea alone reduces the amount of sunburn cells produced under UV light by up to 67 per cent.

Hyaluronic acid is a natural moisturiser that occurs in the skin. It is also a highly effective ingredient in face creams to help prevent moisture loss.

Hydradermie (Previously known as Cathiodermie) is the name of a deep cleansing treatment (for face, eyes and/or back) created by the skincare company, Guinot. It is a unique facial treatment that combines electro-therapy with metal facial rollers to condition the skin, with facial steaming, serious removal of blackheads, and a great facial massage. Ideal for those with normal to oily skins.

Humectants are ingredients in moisturisers which attract moisture from the air and bind them to the surface of the skin.

Ionithermie is a salon treatment for cellulite. It combines a plant and mineral clay-based mask with a gentle electrical current that helps to tone the hips and thighs and improve skin texture.

Iridescent refers to anything that shimmers as it catches the light. Often used when describing make-up that highlights or gives a sheen to the skin.

Kaolin is a white powder which works a little like clay and is used to remove impurities and boost circulation in facial cleansers and masks for normal to oily skins.

Light-reflective (or light-diffusing) describes special pigments in make-up which reflect the light, giving the illusion of younger looking skin.

Lipids are naturally occurring fats in the skin which help to keep it plump, youthful and full of moisture.

Liposomes are high-tech particles which take vital skincare ingredients through the skin and into the epidermis.

Luminous means reflecting the light. Sheer, slightly shimmery face powders can create the illusion of luminous skin because they contain light-reflective particles.

Lycopene is one of the latest antioxidants in skincare, and is believed to be an exceptionally powerful free-radical scavenger. It's found in tomatoes, pink grapefruit, red grapes and watermelon. A deficiency in lycopene is now associated with acne and dermatitis.

Lymphatic system is our internal waste removal system. Lymph, a fluid that circulates around the body, picks up toxins and waste and deposits them in the lymph glands. A build up of waste can result in fatigue and poor circulation.

Matte texture means that skin appears flat and doesn't reflect the light. Matte make-up is usually used to reduce shine on areas such as the T-zone.

Melanin is the natural protective pigment found in skin that turns brown in the sun to form a tan. A tan is our body's natural defence mechanism: it prevents burning and reduces penetration of harmful UV rays. Those with darker skin have more natural melanin and those with red hair and blue eyes have virtually none, so they will never tan.

Microspheres are tiny microscopic particles of an ingredient such as powder. They are used in make-up to make it glide on the skin.

Milia are tiny pearl-like spots that tend to accumulate around the eyes and the cheeks. They are caused by excess sebum becoming trapped underneath the skin, possibly because pores have been clogged by heavy creams. They should always be removed by a qualified beauty therapist.

Nanospheres – see microspheres.

Non-comedogenic – means that the product will not clog pores.

Oestrogen is the female hormone which, among other things, helps to regulate the skin. A good supply of oestrogen usually mean your skin will appear soft and supple, healthy and resilient. Changes in skin are partly due to periodic fluctuations in hormone levels throughout the month or during menopause.

pH refers to acid/alkaline balance. In beauty, it is most often used with reference to the skin. Skin is naturally acidic, with a pH of 4.5 to 5.5. Skin's natural balance can be disturbed by detergents such as soap, which are alkaline.

Pigmentation refers to the skin's colouring. Those with olive or black skin have a dense pigmentation, whereas those with fair skin have little or no natural pigment and appear almost white. Pigmentation problems, such as age spots, birthmarks or vitiligo (loss of pigment), result in patches of pigment which either require treatment (for example with lasers) or concealing camouflage techniques.

Protein contains the 25 essential amino acids which make up the building blocks of the body. Skin is made up of the proteins collagen and elastin, which keep skin soft, supple and youthful. We get protein from fish, meat, lentils, soya and eggs.

Retinol (or retinyls) is the collective term for vitamin A derivatives which are fast gaining popularity as an anti-ageing ingredients in skincare. They are believed to work in a similar way to Retin-A (the renowned acne treatment from America, called Retinova in the UK, which was found to help reduce wrinkles, though it makes skin extremely sun sensitive), but without the irritation. Retinols have been found to help reduce the appearance of age spots, fine lines and smooth the skin's surface. However, their long-term effectiveness is unknown.

Salicylic acid comes from the bark of the willow tree, and has been used for nearly a century as an exfoliator. It is now considered to be the best beta-hydroxy acid (BHA) because it rarely causes irritation and is gentler than AHAs.

Sebum is the correct name for the oil we secrete from our skin and hair.

Semi-permanent is the term given to hair dyes which colour the hair for up to 24 washes, but are not permanent.

SPF stands for Sun Protection Factor and represents the amount of extra time you can stay exposed to the sun without burning. What this means is that if your skin would naturally burn after just 5 minutes in the sun, SPF15 allows you to stay out for 75 minutes (15 x 5).

St John's Wort, or *hypericum*, has been used medicinally for centuries and is widely recognised as an effective natural remedy for mild depression and stress-related problems. It also contains huge amounts of skin regenerating essentials such as flavonoids and tannins.

Titanium oxide is the white pigment used in sunscreens and make-up powders, which acts as a physical block from harmful UV rays.

Toxins are poisons to the system: most notably: alcohol, stress, smoke, pollution, pesticides and food additives. An overload results in poor skin and fatigue, which eventually lead to bowel, bladder, liver and kidney problems.

TEWL (transepidermal water loss) refers to skin's osmotic ability – as water (sweat) comes out, other substances can get in. It is now known that the process of skin absorption is most active at night, making this the best time to use skin treatments.

Ultra-violet rays (UV) are high energy rays of solar radiation which are known to have damaging effects on the skin. UVB (called the Burning ray) penetrates as far as the epidermis and is around all during the summer months; and UVA (the Ageing ray) penetrates deeper into the dermis, and is around all year, whatever the weather. It is vital that skin is protected equally from UVA and UVB.

Zinc oxide is another white pigment, often used in place of titanium dioxide. When finely-milled it makes an excellent sun block and is used in some face powders.

further reference

Useful addresses

Aromatherapy Organisations Council (AOC)

PO Box 19834, London SE25 6WF, Tel: 020 8251 7912

www.aoc.uk.net

Institute of Complementary Medicine (ICM)

PO Box 194, London SE16 1QZ

Society of Teachers of the Alexander Technique

Tel: 020 7284 3338, www.stat.org.uk

The General Osteopathy Council, Osteopathy House, 176
Tower Bridge Road, London SE1 3LU, Tel: 020 7357 6655

For a list of practitioners: www.osteopathy.org.uk

The British Wheel of Yoga, 25 Jermyn Street, Sleaford,
Lincolnshire NG34 7RU, Tel: 01529 306851

The Hale Clinic, 7 Park Crescent, London W1B 1PF,
Tel: 020 7631 0156

Reference Books

The Essence of Aromatherapy by Glenda Taylor (Ryland
Peters & Small, 2000)

The Encyclopedia of Complementary Medicine by Annie
Woodham and Dr. David Peters (Dorling Kindersley, 1997)

Aveda Rituals by Horst Rechelbacher (Ebury Press, 1999)

Bobbi Brown Beauty by Bobbi Brown & Annemarie Iverson
(Collins, 1997).

Eat Fat, Lose Weight by Dr. Ann Louise Gittleman (Keats, 2000)

Before the Change by Dr. Ann Louise Gittleman (HarperSan
Franciso, 2000)

Living Beauty Detox Diet by Dr. Ann Louise Gittleman (Harper-
San Francisco, 2001.

Private make-up lessons

Joy Goodman Hair & Make-up Agency, 3 Lonsdale Road,
London NW6 6RA, Tel: 020 7328 3338. For professional
make-up lessons with a variety of make-up artists (from £200
for two hours).

Hairdressers

Charles Worthington, 7 Percy Street, London W1P 9FB

Tel: 020 7631 1370

Michaeljohn, 25 Albemarle Street, London W1X 4LH

Tel: 020 7409 2956

Nicky Clarke, 130 Mount Street, London W1Y 5HA

Tel: 020 7491 4700

Nationally Approved Salon Campaign (NASC)

Tel: 01302 380006 for your nearest approved hair salon.

Cosmetics companies

BeneFit,Tel: 0901 1130001 (stockists and mail order)

MAC, Tel: 020 7534 9222 (stockists and mail order)

Laura Mercier, Tel: 020 7730 1234 (Harrods mail order)

Guerlain, Tel: 01932 233875 (customer services)

Helena Rubinstein, Tel: 01732 741000 (customer enquiry line)

Yves Saint Laurent, Tel: 01444 255700 (customer services)

Prescriptives, Tel: 0800 525501 (customer services)

index

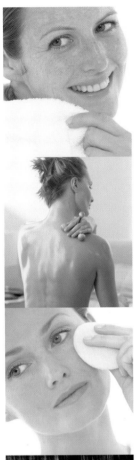

picture credits

Prelims

National Magazine Company Limited Iain Philpott 2; 8
HarperCollins*Publishers* Maureen Barrymore 7 ; Debi Treloar 1, 4

Your Skin

National Magazine Company Limited Roger Eaton 25; Craig Fordham 27; Iain Philpott 12, 17, 20, 23, 31, 33, 43; HarperCollins*Publishers* Maureen Barrymore 11, 19, 28, 34, 44, 46; Derek Lomas 15

Your Body

National Magazine Company Limited Glenn Burnip 50, 55; Wendy Carrig 79; Roger Eaton 49, 72; Craig Fordham 59, 65, 69; Iain Philpott 66, 80, 82; Elizabeth Zeschin 53, 57;
HarperCollins*Publishers* Maureen Barrymore 60, 66 ; Derek Lomas 71

Your Make-up

National Magazine Company Limited Wendy Carrig 86; Yvonne Catterson 99; Richard Dunkley 132; Roger Eaton 92, 130; Annie Johnston 119 (right), 129; Derek Lomas 95, 107, 112; Iain Philpott 119 (left); 121 Polly Wreford 105;
HarperCollins*Publishers* Maureen Barrymore 85, 91, 109; Debi Treloar 89, 97, 101, 103, 111, 117

Your Hair

National Magazine Company Limited Paul Mitchell 143; Tim Winter 155; Annie Johnston 144, 161; Iain Philpott 135, 136, 141, 149, 151, 153, 163, 165;
HarperCollins*Publishers* Debi Treloar 139, 147

Your Mind

National Magazine Company Limited Glenn Burnip 171; Roger Eaton 175, 177; Iain Philpott 167, 172, 178, 180; Elizabeth Zeschin 168

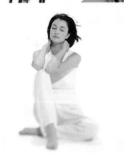

author's acknowledgements

I would especially like to thank Katie Cowan at HarperCollins*Publishers* for her endless patience and support while writing this book; and Vicci Bentley, Ingrid Eames and Emma Dally at *Good Housekeeping* for trusting me to do it in the first place. I would also like to thank Sheena Miller, John Prothero and Kate Hudson for their endless support. And last, but by no means least, my husband Jim and my children Olivia and William who, together, keep me happy and joyful at all times.

Special thanks to Amanda Birch at Michaeljohn's Ragdale Clinic for her anti-ageing facial massage, Alan Herdman for his Pilates session, and Simon Watson for his Daoyin session. And to nutritionist Dr Ann Louise Gittleman, aromatherapist Glenda Taylor, consultant trichologist Glen Lyons at Philip Kingsley, Eve Lom, Janet Filderman, Lynn Rushton at Clarins, make-up artists Ariane Poole, Gillian Buran for Bobbi Brown, Cheryl Phelps-Gardiner, Daniel Sandler, Jillian Veran, Laura Mercier, Maggie Hunt, Olivier Echaudemaison of Guerlain and Roxanne New for their tips and tricks over the years; plus hairdressers Charles Worthington, Denise McAdam, Nicky Clarke and everyone at Michaeljohn.

Many thanks for the loan of cosmetics and make-up props from: BeneFit, Calvin Klein, Charles Worthington, Estée Lauder Companies, Givenchy, Guerlain, and Helena Rubinstein; and to all the beauty PRs who have given me their help.

publishers' acknowledgements

editors	Laura Davies and Michelle Pickering
typesetter	Michelle Pickering
layout designer	Liz Brown
stylist for HarperCollins*Publishers*	Susan Downing
stylist for National Magazine Co. Ltd	Jo Glanville-Blackburn